PRAISE FOR *TRANSFORMED BY BIRTH*

"Britta, you are a master at what you do."

P!NK
Grammy-winning singer-songwriter

"Master teacher, childbirth educator, and doula Britta Bushnell generously shares her most important revelations and strategies in preparing parents for childbirth, and in turn offers them a lifelong gift as they understand themselves anew."

KIMBERLY ANN JOHNSON
author of *The Fourth Trimester: A Postpartum Guide to Healing Your Body, Balancing Your Emotions, and Restoring Your Vitality*

"Britta taught me how to be a birth warrior and I can honestly say, I used Every. Single. Thing I learned in her class during the birth process. I truly don't know how I could have done it without her guidance and the strength of my fellow warrior mamas cheering me on in spirit."

NATALIE ZEA
actress, *The Detour*

"Britta is a gifted teacher, mother, and family advocate who is bringing her soulful passion into this moving offering. *Transformed by Birth* blends her deep understanding of transformational work and her decades supporting birthing families. This book is a gift to pregnant people everywhere."

SHIVA REA
world-renowned yoga teacher

"Having known Britta for decades, I can sincerely recommend the depths of this offering and know that many people will benefit from her wisdom and experience."

SEANE CORN
internationally celebrated yoga teacher, author of *Revolution of the Soul*

"This book is a peace treaty to end the Mommy Wars!"

JOLIE JENKINS
real mom and TV mom on Netflix's *Alexa & Katie*

"I have been a birth doula for over 17 years and have seen first-hand the life-changing transformation women and couples go through as they birth themselves as parents. Thank you, Britta, for writing such an important book! I will be referring this book as a must-read for all!"

LORI BREGMAN
author of *The Mindful Mom-to-Be* and *Mamaste*

"Britta Bushnell has created a unique book that switches the conversation from the minutia of what happens when you have a baby to the identity-changing transformation that takes place when you become a parent. Its pages are filled with simple yet magnificently profound tools to help you truly prepare for the changes that take place in the mythic space of birth, or as Britta poignantly notes, that place 'where you are no longer not a parent and not yet one either.'"

ADRIANA LOZADA
AdvCD(DONA), seasoned doula and host of the *Birthful* podcast

"*Transformed by Birth* offers an unshakable, empathic approach to birth preparation that emphasizes the strengths of openness and resilience. Britta Bushnell's refreshingly original eight ideals for modern preparation guide thinking parents as they traverse two intertwined landscapes: their inner landscape against the backdrop of the medical environment. The book is easy to read, informative, thought-provoking, and uplifting."

PAM ENGLAND
author of *Birthing from Within* and *Ancient Map for Modern Birth*, and
founder of the childbirth training organization Birthing From Within

"Britta brings the most useful information in the most poetic and knowledgeable book. Everything expecting parents need to know in one book."

ANA PAULA MARKEL
past president of DONA International, founder of BINI Birth

"As a midwife, I'm thrilled to finally have a book to confidently recommend for all of my pregnant and parenting clients! With *Transformed by Birth*, Britta Bushnell magically unravels the life-changing experience that is pregnancy, birth, and becoming a parent. This book will blow your heart open and leave you confidently on the threshold of transformation, ready for whatever comes your way as you grow your family."

SARA HOWARD
LM, CPM, IBCLC

"Amidst confusing and divergent opinions around the 'right kind' of birth, this book provides a practical, holistic, and balanced view. While giving information and tools, it also invites the reader to connect with the bigger picture—the transformative power of bringing a child into the world. Britta Bushnell brings her vast experience as a childbirth educator as well as a mother, highlighting and empowering each birthparent's individual experience. Pragmatic yet nuanced, this book educates, expands, and supports each step along the journey from pregnancy to childbirth and beyond. A must read for anyone becoming a parent."

MICHAELA BOEHM
relationship and intimacy expert, author of *The Wild Woman's Way*

"Britta, your words are so needed in the conversation around birth and parenting. My first response to reading this book is 'This is what I want every birthing person to hear.' Your words are full of truth spoken in compassion. I appreciate your honesty about all kinds of births and parenting experiences having the ability to transform a person and removing the shame from the 'non-ideal' birth outcome."

SARAH OBERMEYER
CNM, PhD, WHNP-BC, IBCLC

"When you have an intuition or are aware that pregnancy and delivery may be a profound initiation, soul-changing as well as life-changing, reading *Transformed by Birth* provides insights into questions you didn't know you had, draws upon mythology which in the midst of labor may deepen the experience; and even long after, reading Britta Bushnell's book is likely to bring back the experience with new meaning."

JEAN SHINODA BOLEN
MD, Jungian analyst and author of *Goddesses in Everywoman*
and *Artemis: The Indomitable Spirit in Everywoman*

"*Transformed by Birth* is the much-needed remedy for all of us striving to do motherhood 'right.' Dr. Britta Bushnell delivers an empowering birthing guide for generations to come. This is the parenting book I have been waiting to read!"

ELLIE KNAUS
founder and host of the *Atomic Moms* podcast

Transformed
by Birth

Transformed _by_ Birth

Cultivating

Openness,

Resilience &

Strength for the

Life-Changing

Journey from

Pregnancy to

Parenthood

BRITTA BUSHNELL, PHD

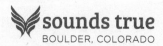

sounds true
BOULDER, COLORADO

Sounds True
Boulder, CO 80306

This book is not intended as a substitute for the medical recommendations of
physicians, mental health professionals, or other health-care providers. Rather, it is
intended to offer information to help the reader cooperate with physicians, mental
health professionals, and health-care providers in a mutual quest for optimal well-
being. We advise readers to carefully review and understand the ideas presented
and to seek the advice of a qualified professional before attempting to use them.

Published 2020

Cover design by Lisa Kerans
Book design by Beth Skelley
Illustrations © 2020 Meghann Stephenson (pages 15, 17, 36, 39, 52, 53, 67, 73,
78, 79, 87, 111, 113, 117, 152, 154, 196, 205, 245, 259, 267)
Illustrations © 2020 Amy Haderer of [M]otherboard (pages 57, 58, 59, 60, 61, 63,
118, 133, 135, 182)

Printed in Canada

Library of Congress Cataloging-in-Publication Data

Names: Bushnell, Britta, author.
Title: Transformed by birth : cultivating openness, resilience, and
    strength for the life-changing journey from pregnancy to parenthood /
    Britta Bushnell, PhD.
Description: Boulder, CO : Sounds True, 2020. | Includes index.
Identifiers: LCCN 2019022888 (print) | LCCN 2019022889 (ebook) |
ISBN   9781683644064 (trade paperback) | ISBN 9781683644132 (ebook)
Subjects: LCSH: Pregnancy. | Childbirth. | Parenting.
Classification: LCC RG525 .B86 2020 (print) | LCC RG525 (ebook) | DDC
    618.2--dc23
LC record available at https://lccn.loc.gov/2019022888
LC ebook record available at https://lccn.loc.gov/2019022889

10 9 8 7 6 5 4 3 2

TO KADEN AND RUMIAH

whose births transformed me—

body, heart, and soul.

Being your mom has been

the greatest joy and

privilege of my life.

TO MY MOM, PAULA,

for loving and supporting me

from day one, including during

my pregnancy, birth, and

postpartum journeys.

Your legacy is woven throughout

the pages of this book.

AND TO ALL PARENTS ON THE

TRANSFORMATIVE JOURNEY

INTO PARENTHOOD.

Everything changed. Every cell, every thought,
every feeling, every heartbeat, every breath, every
sensation, every moment changed forever. Giving birth
is like being put in a crack in the universe, in a space
between being and becoming, between restful stillness
and dynamic growth and change. It was the most
empowering and humbling experience I've ever had.

EMILY

Contents

INTRODUCTION:
No Right Way
to Birth

Like many first-time parents, Katrina[1] immersed herself in books, podcasts, and blogs in preparation for birth. Riveted by a documentary about home birth with midwives, she watched until the end, at which point, she burst into tears.

As Katrina shared this story with me, I thought I understood her feelings. Many parents cry when they see images of birth; they are moved, touched, and inspired by the images that will one day, they hope, be the journey they will take. Listening, I nodded in understanding. Katrina stopped me. "No," she said. "I burst into tears because that was the first time I learned there was a 'right way' to give birth." Katrina felt the pressure of doing birth "right." She thought to herself, "What if I can't do *that*?"

Parents are told by friends and family members the "right way to birth." These include opinions about the right hospital, doctor or midwife, type of pain management—be it medication or hypnosis—and so on. The "right way to birth" ranges from unassisted without any medically trained professionals in attendance to scheduled elective cesarean births. Opinions vary.

Many pregnant parents feel the same agonizing pressure that Katrina felt to do birth "right." The intensity and competition in pregnancy and parenthood rivals that of Olympic events. Upon entering these realms, the focus on getting it right permeates the landscape.

Birth is becoming increasingly polarized; there is more judgment than ever about "right" ways to birth. The polarization evident within our political system, and society as a whole, is strongly represented in the politics, policy, and culture of birth today. Long before the "mommy wars" make their way to playgrounds, they start on the battlefield of birth.

One such polarization of rightness is between the natural and medical birth communities. The battle cries sound something like this: "Birth is natural, not a medical event! Hospitals are for sick people!" to "Birthing at home is irresponsible; what if something were to happen?" and, "We live in the twenty-first century; we don't have to birth like animals!" These binary and polarized camps have done little to ease the mommy wars. Instead, the division is the perfect petri dish to breed judgment—judgment between parents, couples, birth professionals, and even against ourselves.

What can we do instead?

Many people tell pregnant and new parents to "follow their intuition." This can be helpful advice *if* you can easily access your inner wisdom through the fog of so many opinions! It can be difficult to even know where to begin to look for the information you desire.

In need of answers, parents head out in search of evidence that will prove the rightness of one approach or another. Here's the problem: In this era of easily accessed information, we can find "proof" to support whatever we're looking for. Want proof that a hospital birth is *the* safest way to birth? You can find it. Want proof that home birth is *the* safest way to birth? Yep. You can find that too. So, what's a thoughtful and engaged parent to do?

Transformed by Birth does something more than simply arming parents with more information in our already data-inundated culture. It shares wisdom and proven practices to support having a transformational experience of birth, rather than prescribing specific outcomes. In my experience as a birth doula, childbirth educator, and mother, I have seen firsthand and heard many personal stories of births that span the full gamut—from transformative and empowering cesarean births to traumatic unmedicated home births and nearly everything in-between. Outcome alone does not dictate the impact of any given birth. Lots of factors influence the *experience* of birth. And while outcome is important, a singular focus on outcome sidelines both the parents' experience and the transformation that goes far beyond the time of labor and birth, no matter where or how birth happens.

A MEANING-MAKING SPECIES

Humans are a meaning-making species. We crave understanding and meaning, especially around events that defy classification. Those events that reside outside of easy definition, explanation, or clarity often find their home in the language of ritual and myth. Giving birth is one such existential experience.

As animals, survival both as a species and as individuals is of monumental importance; it is *the* thing that matters most. Therefore, surviving birth is tantamount to evolutionary success. But it is not just birth's importance on the evolutionary report card that keeps us engaged with childbirth even when survival is usual. I believe it is childbirth's fundamental character as a rite of passage, as a moment of great transformation created by our biology—our nature—that catapults it into prominence.

There are few moments in a person's life that expose us to such radical change as does the act of giving birth for the first time. Weddings take place with a great deal of ceremony and celebration within our culture, some religions still ritualize coming of age, and death is honored with funerals, but birth, *childbirth*, makes us into something new whether we ritualize it or not. So even while Western culture celebrates birth with few meaningful ceremonies, birth has maintained its place in the overall importance of things because of its evolutionary value, but also because it utterly transforms us, and in the process, shakes the bedrock of our personal world.

When individuals feel vulnerable, what we believe in and what we value most rise to the surface. Facing the act of giving birth, we are tuned in to our innate vulnerability. We strive for security. In contemporary culture, control is worshipped, and as a result, we lean on science, technology, reason, order, and predictability to help us feel safe. Birth practices all along the medical/natural spectrum rally these allies to provide a salve to the underlying anxiety birth produces. Childbirth and new parenthood cause us to question who we are and what we value. Existential anxiety is to be expected.

It's normal to crave understanding and control. Mystery and uncertainty are not comfortable sensations for most of us, and modern advancements have reduced our familiarity with these feelings. In today's society, few experiences reside outside of intellectual understanding and mechanistic control. Gone are the days where few things were understood scientifically, where explanation was handled almost exclusively by the myths and stories of a people, where healing was addressed ritualistically, and mystery was a daily companion.

As a species, we've come a long way. We understand so much more about how the world works. No longer is a story about a goddess mourning her daughter's time in the Underworld relied upon to explain changing seasons. (While this particular story is of Greek origin, each culture had, or still has, its own stories to explain elements of the world that were not understood.) Now we understand the tilting axis of the Earth in its orbit around the sun. In some ways, we have replaced one story with another. It could be said that science has become the most widespread human mythology. It has an explanation for everything, or at least we like to believe it does. Science has soothed much of the anxiety that arises in the face of mystery.

But mystery still exists.

Childbirth and parenthood continue to challenge our efforts to control; science cannot remove all uncertainty. These areas continue to challenge us with their mysterious ways, their chaotic rhythms, and their constantly changing nature. Childbirth and parenthood defy mechanization. Few reliable scientific formulas exist in these realms. *A* plus *B* does not always, or even often, equal *C*.

Technology alone cannot remove us from the mysteries of birth, nor of parenthood. When parents become aware of birth as an instrument of great transformation and power, reverence, humility, and respect are brought back to this ultimate human experience.

Simply put: *birth matters.*

MY STORY

I've been working in the field of childbirth for over twenty years. For me, birth is a rite of passage—a threshold into vibrant awareness and existential crisis and a catalyst for profound change. Unlike most birth professionals, I do not consider birth itself to be my primary passion. The thread that weaves several seemingly unrelated fields to form the tapestry of my work is a passion for growth and transformation.

When I was eight years old, my stepmom gave birth to my little brother. While in labor, as her contractions came and went, she taught me gin rummy. When a contraction started, we would pause the game so she could focus until the contraction subsided. I didn't know then that this experience would be the first of many times I would sit with a parent during labor.

In 1999, I was pregnant with my first child and teaching prenatal yoga classes at the now-famous YogaWorks in Santa Monica, California. Several times a week I led a group of pregnant women through ninety minutes of stretches, breathing exercises, and visualizations, helping them to leave the class grounded and "in their bodies." After birth, parents would often come back to the classes, and time after time these new moms would exclaim, "*My* birth was *really* intense!"

I began to understand that I was somehow communicating that to do birth "yogically," parents should be able to simply breathe, relax, and meditate through labor as we had done in class. I never mentioned pain, hard work, or effort. Without realizing it, I denied the very real possibility of facing hardships in labor or parenthood. I was unwittingly rendering these birthing parents underprepared for labor and birth.

By that point, I had given birth to my first child, an experience that was intense, unexpected, and powerful. I knew personally that yogic breathing and relaxation were helpful for birth and parenthood, but also that these experiences required far more.

I began hunting for a more complete way to support parents on the journey from pregnancy to parenthood. This quest led me to take a class early in 2002 with Pam England, author of the book *Birthing from Within* and director of the organization Birthing From Within. What she was doing with birth preparation felt revolutionary, personal, and spiritually rich. I was hooked!

Pam became my mentor, a colleague on my journey as a childbirth professional, for a time my business partner, and ultimately, a trusted friend. The Birthing From Within approach and my close relationship with Pam have highly influenced my work, my life, and with her blessing, this book.

Late in the summer of 2009, in search of the next step along my career path, I saw mention of a graduate degree program in mythology. I was pulled deeper, salivating at the course titles and reading every description. This program focused not just on the great stories themselves but also on the psychological impact they have on us as humans. That fall, I enrolled in graduate school in pursuit of a doctorate in mythological studies.

In grad school, I vowed to branch out beyond childbirth. But it didn't matter which course I took, be it Hinduism, Fairy Tales, The God Complex, or Ritual, I couldn't help but hear themes related to childbirth. As I explored topics for my dissertation, the loudest voice within me kept calling me to write about birth. For over two years, I researched, studied, and wrote my dissertation titled, *Forceps and Candles: Cultural Myths in American Childbirth*, which turned out to be the research phase of this book.

Over the past twenty years, I also raised two kids: one has been successfully launched into college, and the other is not far behind. I have learned a huge amount in the process of parenthood. My children are profound teachers. I've made mistakes—learned from some and repeated others. Parenting is a practice that humbles me, exhausts me, and enlivens me. It continues to teach me the importance of openness, resilience, and strength . . . *daily*! As does my relationship with my husband, Brent. Parenthood challenges our communication, our power dynamic, our sex life, our roles as co-parents, and our individual and professional identities as well as our identity as a couple. We have worked to make tending to our relationship a priority. We have learned and adopted several tools and practices that have profoundly supported our partnership throughout our more than twenty-five years as a couple and almost twenty years as co-parents. As couples began bringing their relationship struggles to me for help, I started sharing these tools and practices with them. I include a few of the best of these in this book.

The process of writing this book has been somewhat similar to the process of becoming a parent. As I write, I feel connected to you with all the fear, excitement, expectation, and attachment that come with a process of creation. Nearly every word I wrote here about birth, bravery, facing the unexpected, and continuing to move forward anyway, I had to take to heart myself in the writing process. Birthing comes in many forms, and openness, resilience, and strength are needed for all of them.

AUTHOR'S NOTE

This book is for parents. Parents come in many forms and arrive at the point of parenthood down different paths. This book is for those sharing the journey with a partner and/or a co-parent as well as for those going solo by choice or by situation. It is for gay parents, heterosexual parents, transgender parents, gender fluid parents, pregnant parents, adoptive parents, surrogate parents, parents who wanted to be parents, and those surprised by the prospect of becoming parents. It is my hope that if you are in a partnership, you'll read this book together and if you are solo, you'll share sections of this book with those you consider part of your support team on your journey into parenthood.

As this book is intended for parents, not just mothers, I use the term parents throughout the book. Sometimes I need to differentiate between the parent birthing and the supporting parent. When that happens, I will most often refer to the one who will be giving birth as the birthing parent and the other parent as the partner. When I share stories about other parents, and I know their chosen parental name, I use it. Whichever way you choose to identify—whether it's as mama, mom, mother, mommy, ima, mum, ama, father, papa, dad, daddy, dada, apu, pa, or one of a million other possibilities—is wonderful!

I am assuming that you are becoming a parent and that's why you picked up this book about the transformative journey from pregnancy to parenthood. Join me as we explore and prepare for the wild ride that is the metamorphic transformation into parenthood.

PART I

Preparing
for the
Journey

Birth as a
Meaning-Making
Experience

I have already stated that I view birth as a rite of passage, but what exactly does that mean? What is a rite of passage?

Rites of passage are *meaningful* transformational experiences that alter a person's knowing of who they are. They usually have an element of struggle or some level of discomfort or involve facing an ordeal. A rite of passage takes an initiate out of their familiar identity of daily life and thrusts them into something new, often stressful, and possibly threatening. Through these unfamiliar challenges, existential questions about the meaning of life, higher purpose, and the nature of God are made central.

Rites of passage are sometimes divided into three phases. Arnold van Gennep, who coined the phrase *rites of passage*, identified these three parts as separation, transition, and reincorporation.[1] Bruce Lincoln's three-part structure involved enclosure, metamorphosis, and emergence. He developed this structure after observing rites of passage given to young women.[2] Lincoln's three phases mirror the journey of the caterpillar entering the cocoon and coming out a butterfly, a metaphor I use often for the process of the transformation into parenthood.

Initiation rites given to young people coming into adulthood often test the individual in physical, emotional, and spiritual ways. These initiatory ordeals test courage, commitment, and endurance. Even though success is typical, these rites of passage contain risk and often great struggle. It is by coming through the fire of initiation that the child self dies and the adult self is born. Can you see the ways this mirrors the process of labor into birth for many parents?

To face the unknown inherent in birthing, including your own animal nature, you must learn to embrace that which cannot be understood or processed rationally or learned through purely intellectual means. For this, you must practice *letting go*. This is not to be understood as resigning yourself to victimization or innocently handing over power or control to another but rather being openly passionate and dispassionate, engaged but not attached, at the same time.

While not the only way, the process of birthing is the primary way that a person becomes a parent, particularly with a first birth. This passage takes an individual from one social and biological state into another. But for birth to be a rite of passage it requires more than the act of giving birth, it requires a different relationship to the *meaning* of the process. To view birth as an initiatory process is to understand and even *value* the unpredictability and uncontrollability of even the best-laid plans. Fear of this "not-knowing" aspect of birthing is central to preparation for birth as a rite of passage rather than a shadow component to be avoided. Birth as an initiatory journey embraces the challenges and ordeals along the way, as part of the very path the new parents will travel.

MYTH, RITUAL, AND CHILDBIRTH

Current birthing practices focus on the outcome and location of birth: surgical or vaginal, medicated or unmedicated, hospital or home. Little focus is placed on the body, mind, spirit, and relationships of the human beings involved.

After an unwanted cesarean, well-meaning professionals and friends often say, "Be happy! Your baby is healthy." Comments of this sort place the emphasis on outcome, ignoring or sidelining the emotional confusion often present at the birth of a desired baby through the means of an unwanted surgery. Similarly, the more radical natural birth proponents often see the inability to birth at home or without drugs as failure, as if the only thing that matters is the fulfillment of the natural birth image. The loss of an ideal held so dearly can traumatize or victimize birthing parents. Focus on outcome ignores the importance of the transformations that go beyond the physical expulsion of a baby from its parent's body.

When focused on the outcome of birth alone—vaginal or surgical, medicated or natural, home or hospital—it's easy to lose sight of the existential experience of *giving birth* that does not fit neatly in any binary box. We have to expand beyond the black-and-white classifications and outcome-focused myopia to a more colorful palette that includes the multiplicity of experiences inherent in giving birth. We must shift from focusing exclusively on a healthy baby/healthy mother as the only factors in determining a successful birth to a more pluralistic focus that includes a healthy baby/healthy family *and* a meaningful transformative experience.

Truly holistic preparation includes the mind, spirit, body, and intimate relationships, the combination of which resists classification and might best be described as mythic. Holistic, mythic birth preparation includes physical, mental, emotional, and spiritual components that support the understanding that giving birth is a rite of passage.

This type of preparation defies dualistic categorization. It does not prescribe an approach that says, "your body knows how to birth," nor does it see pain as a problem requiring remedy or something that must be suffered through. A mythic approach to birth prepares parents for that which lies beyond duality. Childbirth preparation of this type dances on the delicate ground of espousing no privileged experiences. The challenges birth brings are yours to face as part of your unique initiation into parenthood.

Contrary to what some birth activists propose, birth cannot be fixed by simply returning to previous ways of thinking when birth was only wild and untamed, where the most dangerous thing in a woman's life was the possibility of dying in childbirth. This gamble is no longer required of most parents, at least not as often. While there is certainly still a gamble, the stakes fall more in our favor. In today's culture there is a medical safety net that can often catch us when nature's answer to birth is death.

Following your nature now includes navigating situations when nature asks too high a price. Birthing as a rite of passage is surrendering to oneness with nature—your nature—and letting go when that nature includes the advancements offered through science and technology. Who beyond the individual parent can know for certain what it means to follow their nature?

In today's birth culture, dancing in these flowered and thorny fields of nature and technology requires a different type of preparation, one that is as multidimensional as birth itself. It requires more heart and less intellectualization, more real power and less victimization, more openness and less idealization, more myth and fewer statistics, more moderation and less extremism. Parents preparing for birth need more of what the culture lacks. You need to move toward the mystery, not because it is better than science, but because there is less of it present in modern culture and, it could be argued, because birthing is the most intense mysterious human experience next to death.

ENTERING INTO SACRED SPACE

When we enter the world of birth, we step across the threshold from the mundane to the sacred. Pregnancy and birth are a space between worlds—a liminal space—a place where you are no longer *not* a parent and not yet one either. This betwixt and between is sacred space within which powerful and profound events occur—often uninvited. There was a time when pregnant women would actually enter a different physical space—a special lodge, confinement room, or birthing hut—to mark their time moving from the mundane world to the sacred. While this sort of noticeable separation no longer makes sense in the lives of modern parents, the profundity of pregnancy and birth as a place between worlds is no less potent. As a modern-day parent, if you desire a space of special honoring, you have to create it for yourself while continuing to engage with the everyday world of normal life.

When using words like *sacred* and *transcendent* in discussions about birth, it's easy to get the impression that the process is lofty in a way that is purely beautiful or enchanting. And while birth can be both beautiful and enchanting, it is often far grittier and earthy than *transcendent* and *sacred* imply to modern ears. There is something about birth that, while deeply spiritual and meaningful, is actually grounded in raw and gritty "now-ness." Ancients understood the sacred to include these darker aspects, but as modern people, we've changed the ideas of sacred and transcendent to be photo-ready. When people think about birth as a spiritual or transcendent experience, they conjure images up of flowing nightgowns, burning candles, and the feeling of reverence that stunning art, some religious services, and epic nature can invoke. In reality, what is truly spiritual is often far messier than social media-ready images imply. Birth, while transcendent, otherworldly, spiritual, and profound, is actually intense hard work that tests our ideas of what "spiritual" looks like and means. Birth exposes the sacred through the muck, mud, and hardship of something so profoundly animalistic that it makes us into something entirely new. This otherworldly place where great transformation happens is the sacred space of birth.

THE MESSY MIDDLE

The current dominant approaches to childbirth—both medical and natural—often bypass the process of transformation that turns an individual into a parent and a couple into a family. This skip is akin to a caterpillar strapping on wings to declare itself a butterfly! Without the metamorphosis within the cocoon, there is no butterfly.

What happens in the cocoon is not glamorous. This process is often completely hidden to the public eye and lacks a place of prominence within society. We read about the hungry caterpillar who eats and eats and, after a single page dedicated to the time spent in the cocoon, becomes a beautiful butterfly. From a cultural perspective, the journey into parenthood seems to mirror this storybook process. We spend months becoming the big full-bellied pregnant parent only to expect to pop out on the other side of birth as a fully formed parent butterfly ready to spread its wings and fly.

As social worker and author Brené Brown says, you can't skip the "messy middle."[3] In the process of becoming a parent, the messy middle is the cocoon phase of transfiguration where the identity is completely reconfigured into a person who is also a parent. First, there is a dissolving, and then, a rebuilding. This transfiguration takes place in the cocoon of pregnancy, birth, and postpartum. It is rarely talked about and is certainly messy. Ultimately, wings are formed, and flight becomes possible, but the destination is not the journey, and the journey matters. Transformation requires more than physically birthing a baby.

This book is like an X-ray into what happens in the cocoon and how to prepare for it. Becoming a parent is a metamorphosis into a new identity that did not exist before. The time spent in the cocoon offers a rich and powerful opportunity for deep personal exploration and growth.

GATHER 'ROUND THE FIRE

If you walked into my teaching space for a childbirth class, you would see mythologically themed art on the walls, a circle of chairs, and a centerpiece on the floor filled with props for teaching—statues, symbols, toys, anatomical models, and at the center, a candle or two. While these props help keep classes engaging, my primary teaching tools are imagery, storytelling, symbolism, and metaphor. These tools are more necessary than any physical prop, and I am still able to share them with you in written form. While it might seem strange at first to learn about childbirth through metaphor and myth, there is science behind this method.

The Ancient Technology of Storytelling

Imagine that you live thousands of years ago, back when the majority of the population lived in tribal societies. Your community sleeps in easily transportable homes, in caves, or out in the open. You and your family subsist on what can be hunted or gathered. And when it gets dark, you gather for warmth and protection around a fire. In a circle around the fire are your friends and family. Within the captivating light of the fire and circle of community, stories are shared. These stories are meant to entertain as well as to teach about and prepare for life's important events. Whether it's to ready themselves for a hunt, relocation, harvest, ceremony, or battle, your people use stories to share the process of preparation communally. Mesmerized by the

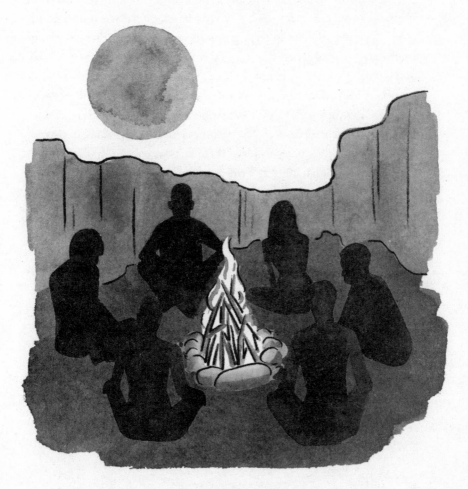

intoxication of the fireside scene, you are receptive to the stories and listen attentively to the teller. You become one with the story and its characters, entering the story as if it were *your* story.

For millennia people have gathered around fires to hear stories in front of a blazing hearth or while camping. Stories shared around a fire cast a powerful and engaging spell upon the listener.

But over the years, storytelling and metaphor have been relegated predominantly to the realm of movies and novels and dismissed as mere entertainment. Their value as preparation and education has diminished. Contemporary culture places a high value on logic, reason, and scientific facts, but the inverse is true of story, imagination, and instinct, as these have been devalued as less reliable, trustable, or true. Modern culture has encyclopedic levels of information available at a moment's notice. Smartphones often live in our pockets. If information alone were the only necessary key to a successful birthing or parenting journey, birth and parenthood today would be wildly successful—*all of the time*. This is simply not the case.

According to Daniel Pink, author of *A Whole New Mind: Why Right-Brainers Will Rule the Future*, "When facts become so widely available and instantly accessible, each one becomes less valuable. What begins to matter more is the ability to place these facts in context and to deliver them with emotional impact."[4] This is where using story comes in. Story invites us to return to the fireside, where learning and preparation capture the imagination, where we enjoy and engage with a story as a whole person, where we enter the story ourselves and use that experience to gain wisdom. Learning through story doesn't just teach us what we need to know but also what to do with that newly found wisdom.

We wrap ourselves in stories and mythology to help us understand who we are and what is important. Stories, myths, and metaphors illuminate aspects of life that defy explanation, including birth. Through great stories, we are able to communicate about existential and transcendent experiences that are otherwise indescribable. Great stories let us face huge unfathomable events and imagine ourselves within them confronting the dragons of our unconscious. Stories teach us how to navigate challenges by using what Jonathan Gottschall calls in his book, *The Storytelling Animal*, "a powerful and ancient virtual reality technology that simulates the big dilemmas of human life."[5] Through story, we get to try things on, practice, and learn to solve problems before we ever have to face something of that sort in real life. Story does all of this under cover of the ever-watchful rational brain.

The value of storytelling as a means for learning is becoming more scientifically understood as neuroscience advances. It turns out story and metaphor are far stickier than mere facts and figures. We remember stories; we forget facts. One theory about this phenomenon is that stories engage our emotions. The brain releases dopamine when emotionally aroused, and this chemical enhances memory.[6] Neuroeconomist Paul Zak demonstrated in his studies "that character-driven stories with emotional content result in a better understanding of the key points . . . and enable better recall of these points weeks later."[7] As Daniel Pink says, "Stories are easier to remember—because in many ways, stories are how we remember."[8] Stories stay in your memory longer. Period.

There's more. Storytelling specialist Doug Stevenson says that "stories are memorable because of the images and emotions contained in them. The lesson of the story sticks because it's embedded in an image. The image isn't a still picture; it's a motion picture, a movie . . . Your brain remembers pictures first. It then remembers the emotional context, and finally, it remembers language."[9] Images are more easily remembered, whereas statistics and facts are often forgotten.

Myth, Metaphor, and the Birthing Brain

There are even more reasons for using stories to learn about birth and new parenthood. I explained above how stories, myth, and metaphors are generally memorable and stay within our accessible memory far better than charts and lists. But this is even *more applicable* within the hormonally charged brain of a laboring or postpartum person. Thanks to the hormonal flood in labor, the neocortex—where logic, rational thinking, and language rule—is subdued. Birth hormones stimulate the older parts of the brain that are more instinctual, primal, and ani- malistic, where symbols and imagery have greater lasting power (we'll discuss labor hormones more in chapter 5).

When a story engages us to the point where we emotionally reso-nate with the characters, we begin to empathize, and a process called "narrative transportation" occurs. Oxytocin, the hormone primarily responsible for labor contractions and bonding, is also "responsible for empathy and narrative transportation."[10] Great stories produce a release of oxytocin in the brain. Oxytocin exists in high quantities during labor, birth, and lactation, and it has been shown that memory is enhanced when learning and recall happen in the same emotional state.[11] An oxytocin-induced state is present when we receive stories *and* when we experience key childbearing moments. This well-matched state enhances recall.

This book takes all of this into account and is loaded with powerful tools of the imaginal realm based on years of experience witnessing the impact of story, myth, and metaphor on expectant parents. You will come across myths as stories and mythological entities as metaphors. You will read stories shared by parents and stories from my own life. And you will experience lots of metaphors—some are visual, while others are whimsically woven into the text.

Some of the images shared will inspire joy; others may challenge or even elicit fear. Mine is not a style of story sharing that is restricted to only those stories of magical births that create a lopsided image of reality. The full range of experiences and emotions are welcome here. Birth and new parenthood require you to get gritty, face things you find distasteful, *and* find your way through them anyway. Expanding your capacity to navigate discomfort is key to the rite of passage you are embarking upon. My years of working with expectant families have shown me that you are strong enough to face the challenges, fully experience the joys, and open to new possibilities. Let's dive in!

2

Start Where
You Are

Congratulations! You're having a baby!

This simple phrase makes it seem as if there is a single experience of becoming pregnant and readying for birth. But this is not the case. Some people are surprised by an unexpected pregnancy, others struggle for years to get pregnant, and others traverse through multiple pregnancy losses unsure if *this time* the pregnancy will stick.

Throughout my years of teaching classes, I have heard many different paths parents have taken to arrive to the point where they are in my class preparing for birth. Every story is unique. There are young parents, as well as older parents. There are married, partnered, single, heterosexual, and gay parents. There are parents new to the area with no extended family nearby and those who have always lived with their parents. There are couples who have known one another for a very short time and those who were childhood sweethearts. No two parents have had the same experiences influencing their lives and leading them to this moment in time.

Sometimes, the stories are of surprise, disbelief, and even shock. I remember the first time a couple shared with the class that they barely knew one another as they, very unexpectedly, got pregnant on their first date! Since then, I've heard similar stories several times. They are often punctuated by a decision about what to do with this highly unexpected pregnancy.

Then there are the stories of struggle. These are the heartbreaking tales of challenge, infertility, and loss. Over the years, I've seen the desire to share and speak the truth of fertility struggles grow. Slowly, we're moving this previously taboo topic out of the shadows and breaking the silence around miscarriage and infertility, creating instead a culture of compassion and tenderness that allows these previously whispered conversations the airtime they deserve.

And then, of course, there are the couples who consciously decide to start a family and become and stay pregnant easily and without complication. There is no one single path, just as there is no universal way to birth.

The entire journey from becoming pregnant through parenthood is an opportunity for deep personal discovery. It's time to reflect on your relationship to pregnancy and birth. Use the following questions as inspiration for journaling or meditative self-inquiry. Or, if you are in a relationship, let these questions launch an engaging conversation with your partner. Whatever way you use these questions, move slowly through them, allowing time for reflections and insights to arise.

- **How did you arrive at this point?** How did you become pregnant? What did you learn as a result of your path to pregnancy? Look for life lessons you've either gleaned or could extract from what you've experienced.

- **Did you experience infertility, pregnancy loss, or have to terminate an earlier pregnancy on the journey to this pregnancy?** If so, how did you get through the challenging moments? How did you keep going? How have those experiences influenced your connection to this pregnancy?

- **How has your experience with pregnancy in the past (your own or witnessing others' pregnancies) impacted you in this pregnancy?** Pay attention to the messages you have received throughout your life about pregnancy. Did you have experiences with your own parents during their pregnancy with one of your siblings, or was a close friend pregnant before you, or did you know someone who became pregnant very young? How do any or all of these experiences inform your relationship to being pregnant? My stepmom had six babies from the time I was eight to when I was twenty-four. Watching her navigate pregnancy six times influenced what I believed to be true about it. Those beliefs surfaced when I became pregnant with my firstborn.

- **What cultural messages have you received about pregnancy?** Culture can mean a lot of different things. For example, I have a friend who grew up believing that pregnancy makes you fragile, while another saw pregnancy as the highest form of health. The culture I grew up in was one highly informed by my mother who worked as a pregnancy counselor from when I was in late elementary school through high school. Conversations around our dinner table often involved my mom's concern for someone she had met that day at work who was very young and unexpectedly pregnant. In addition to these family conversations, sex education was all about birth control and reducing accidental pregnancy. Like many people, I grew up believing we had to be vigilant because pregnancy could happen *very* easily. What messages did you get about pregnancy?

- **What is your relationship status and how does it influence how you feel about being pregnant?** What about your relationship status works for you? How would you like it to be better? What's one small step you could take toward improving it? If you are in a relationship, how does your partner feel about this pregnancy? How does their experience of this pregnancy influence you?

- **What do you believe is the role of a partner in pregnancy, labor, birth, and new parenthood?** Without lots of consciousness, we create expectations about the role we want our partner to play during pregnancy, labor, birth, and new parenthood. I often hear birthing parents bemoaning the lack of involvement on the part of their partner. They want them to build the crib, help pick out the best car seat, come up with names, attend prenatal appointments with their health-care provider, and read books about birth. While all of these are perfectly normal expectations, we get into trouble when our expectations are not explored and expressed.

  On the flip side, partners may expect that the birthing parent simply "knows best" about baby-related things. Exploring expectations about what you imagine your partner will and won't do is a great way to reduce the fuel that enflames resentment. Plus, practicing communication of this type develops skills useful far into your co-parenting relationship.

- **What cultural messages have you received about labor and birth?** Have you witnessed a birth in person before? Maybe you've witnessed hundreds as a birth professional or witnessed the family pet giving birth, or maybe you've never seen a birth other than those depicted on TV or in movies. What have these experiences taught you about birth? What are your expectations about birth as a result of these messages?

  No one enters pregnancy or birth without messages embedded within their unconscious about what being pregnant and giving birth are like. These messages inform much of how we engage with pregnancy and birth. Bringing them to the surface helps us become familiar with the bedrock beneath the decisions we make and expands our understanding of the emotions evoked along the path into parenthood. We are influenced by many personal factors unique to particular life experiences, as well as biological influences and unconscious conditioning embedded within the broader cultural context.

THE CULTURE OF CONTEMPORARY CHILDBIRTH

Contemporary society has created and is guided by fundamental cultural *myths*—what I refer to in this book as "ideals." Beliefs, behaviors, and policy around how we give birth are inextricably intertwined within the powerful net cast by these ideals. The idea of there being a *single* culture is overly simplified, and any attempt to streamline something as complex as guiding ideals runs the risk of heavy oversimplification. And yet, notwithstanding these risks, categorizing these themes has brought value to those I've worked with and has added greater understanding about giving birth in today's cultural climate.

I believe there are many ideals at play within Western culture that impact the transformative journey through childbirth and into parenthood. And as I research and continue to work with both parents and fellow birth professionals, I keep identifying more that I want to add to this list. I have limited my exploration within this book to these eight:

1. Desire for control and the need for certainty

2. Veneration of information and technology

3. Reverence for ordered culture over wild nature

4. Vilification of pain

5. Glorification of independence

6. Adherence to innocence

7. Denial of death

8. Quest for perfection and exceptionalism

To focus entirely on these ideals keeps us spiraling within the problems that stem from them. Instead, I will address the cultural ideals *and* ways parents-to-be can move beyond the bonds imposed by them. In this way, the desire for control is tempered by an openness to the unexpected. Intellectual knowledge along with the veneration of technology is transformed into embodied wisdom. Reverence for a well-ordered society is balanced with awe for the wild nature of birth. Innocence matures and pain's alchemical role in growth is better understood. The "going it alone" message of independence gives way to partnership and community. Identity death is valued as a necessary stage for rebirth, and the quest for perfection is grounded in humility and sufficiency. Taking the perspective of birth as a rite of passage, an initiatory journey of transformation, means that positive birth experiences are not exclusively dependent upon idyllic births or an improved birth culture.

That is not to say that improvements in the state of current birth practices aren't needed. Real problems exist that no understanding of birth as a rite of passage can fix. It is now mostly agreed that the national average for births by cesarean is too high.[1] Additionally, studies addressing the quality of care available to birthing families and mortality rates by race and socioeconomic class demonstrate the devastating reality of massive inequality and the effects of systemic racism.[2] And massive policy and cultural change is needed to support families in the postpartum period as well. These are real problems that demand action whether birth is reenvisioned and prepared for as a rite of passage or not.

My focus is not on what needs to change "out there" in the realm of cultural birthing practices. Instead, I propose that changing the way you prepare for birth and becoming a parent can improve your *experience* of giving birth regardless of how you birth. Engaging your mind, body, spirit, and relationships in the preparatory process for birth as a rite of passage changes not just the experience of birth but also the successful and meaningful transformation into parenthood.

PART II

Birth *and* Culture

Eight Cultural Ideals

Prepare to Be
Unprepared

Billy, a doctor, and Sharon, a business owner, took my classes several years ago. They showed up to the first class and announced that they were open to learning about childbirth, but they planned to "get the epidural" as soon as they got to the hospital. They had a plan. Labor, birth, and all that messiness were not part of it. Contractions would start, and they would go to the hospital, get an epidural, and have a baby. Done. As often happens, birth had other plans.

Neela liked her doctor, a woman she had seen as her gynecologist for several years, and had established what she referred to as a good relationship. Neela and her husband, Tom, were planning an unmedicated hospital birth. Neela planned to work up until their baby was born and return to work after a two-month maternity leave. Their transition into parenthood was organized, scheduled, and predictable. As a financial *planner*, Neela was well versed in creating a nicely organized *plan* for this next big event in their lives. Neela and Tom's entire lives had been supported by their well-honed control skills; why should giving birth be any different?

Like so many, neither of these two births happened as the parents planned or expected.

THE DESIRE FOR CONTROL
AND THE NEED FOR CERTAINTY

Of course, we want control and certainty. As modern-day humans, we gain comfort from predictability. When we know what to expect and can plan our approach or dictate outcomes, we feel that all is right with the world. On the other hand, when events are unpredictable, out of our control, or uncertain, we become anxious, nervous, and often feel off-kilter. Our natural response to the difficult feelings brought on by facing unpredictable events is to seek methods for creating more control and certainty.

While there are ways to improve your chances of pregnancy and labor events going well or close to your hopes for them, childbirth simply does not work like a predictable, well-oiled machine. Even with the best-laid plans, pregnancy, birth—and certainly parenthood—can throw us curveballs when we least expect them.

Childbirth is more than a biological event or a psychological event or a relational event or a medical event. It is all those things and much more. Childbirth is a transformational experience that alters a parent's knowing of who they are. It is an epic journey, one that takes parents to the dark woods of their own powerful undoing. Believing in the illusion that one can control birth robs the process of the benefit that a true rite of passage affords: aiding in the successful transformation of one's identity.

Over the two decades I've worked with birthing families, I have seen highly educated, engaged, powerful, and purposeful individuals craft elaborate expectations for their labor, birth, and postpartum period. They do all the "right" things to make the birth go as planned, to follow the path they desire, and still surprises arise. It doesn't matter if those plans call for an idyllic home birth or a planned hospital birth with pharmaceutical pain support or even a scheduled birth by cesarean . . . no one escapes all unexpected events on the journey into and through parenting.

And yet, new methods to control events and create certainty in the childbearing year surface all the time. Anxiety, often at the forefront of pregnancy, makes parents susceptible to the latest tonic—be it truly magical or merely inert ingredients dressed up in a fancy bottle. Still, we buy the potion, attend the hottest birthing or parenting classes, and continue to seek relief from our anxiety, hoping to find the secret to birthing without pain or to getting our baby to sleep well.

No such perfect anxiety-relieving remedies can remove all uncertainty and create definitive control. While we can influence many contributing factors in our lives, ultimate control and certainty are impossible. What we need most are not methods for better control but rather more resilience and adaptability for when events surprise, challenge, or disappoint us.

Perhaps the most pervasive aspect of the contemporary cultural paradigm is the belief that we have control over our lives. Core Western values such as liberty, the pursuit of happiness, and autonomy are all tied into the concept of control. Each of the following chapters addresses specific cultural ideals, all of which are tangled in an intricate dance with the illusion of control.

Before the advent of modern science, people had little faith that things were within human control. They looked to the gods, stories, and faith in divine power to explain and give comfort in the tossing sea of mortal uncertainty. Perhaps what has changed is not that we humans wish to have control over our lives but the means by which we attempt to acquire that power.

Compared to our forebears' prayers to supernatural powers, the technological age has provided incredible amounts of hope that ultimate control is an attainable goal. The scientific method of testing hypotheses through repeatable experiments created a greater sense of control and certainty. We now have more power over our lives than ever. We can fly through the air, cutting travel time to a fraction of what it was a century ago. We communicate across the globe in an instant. Life-saving medical equipment is increasing our longevity and reducing pain and suffering. We can see into the womb and in so doing detect fetal malformations and determine the gender of our unborn child as no amulets or pendulums ever could. Agricultural advancements make crop yields higher than anything achievable through the most reverent of ritual dances. The possibility of completely controlling our environment and our lives seems ever more attainable. We believe in the possibility that *we are actually in control.*

And yet our physical bodies continue to pose a problem. Even with scientific advancements in areas of technology, physiology, biomedicine, and neuroscience, the body is hardly the perfect student. Instead, the body is wild. We continue to wrestle with the body in an attempt to bend it to our will. And still, the body resists. There is no strategy to wholly control it; we cannot create the perfect vitamin concoction, discover an infallible diet, design the ideal living environment, or develop technology capable of "unwilding" the nature of our bodily condition. Childbirth brings the uncontrollable reality of our bodies into sharp relief.

Maybe childbirth is more predictable, ordered, and controlled than it once was. Parents and babies are surviving birth at rates that would have astounded our ancestors. So what then is the problem with attempting to control childbirth?

Control is a problem because it is ultimately an illusion.

OPENING TO THE UNBIDDEN

Childbirth and parenthood test our belief in control and certainty in profound ways. Children live outside of our bodies and yet feel very much like a part of us. Other people, outside events, and our own reactions and behavior collectively create the reality of any situation. In the best case, we only have control over our personal reactions and behavior and even that is questionable. It is not possible to control all aspects of one's life. We contribute to the events of our lives but cannot entirely determine what happens to us. We can influence, but not control.

In his article "The Case Against Perfection," Michael Sandel writes:

> We choose our friends and spouses at least partly on the basis of qualities we find attractive. But we do not choose our children. Their qualities are unpredictable, and even the most conscientious parents cannot be held wholly responsible for the kind of children they have. That is why parenthood, more than other human relationships, teaches what the theologian William F. May calls an "openness to the unbidden."[1]

By definition, something that is unbidden has not been invited. Parenthood teaches us to be open to that which we do not ask for, desire, or control—sometimes kicking and screaming—until we either learn to be more open or continue the struggle. We spend a lot of time, energy, and money attempting to selectively invite only those aspects of labor and birth we deem positive through our individual and cultural lenses.

The opposite of desiring control and needing certainty is a practice of openness to the unbidden. I am not saying that we should abandon all efforts toward a meaningful birth experience or forsake all attempts to raise good and kind children. No, there is a time and place for learning, preparing, and honing our skills, *and* there is a time to let go and ride the waves of the moment as they come.

To be open to the unbidden is letting things be in their uncertainty and mystery without attempting to shape them into another form through an inflexible force of will. This is not to be understood as resigning into victimhood or innocently handing over power and control to another, but rather being openly passionate and dispassionate, engaged but not attached at the same time. Actually doing this is no easy task, but with practice, we can become more familiar with uncertainty and mystery. In the exercises sprinkled throughout this chapter (as well as throughout this book), I will share ways to develop more courage and comfort in the face of the unknown.

Many methods to control and order the unpredictable aspects of birth do so by attempting to turn the body into a predictable machine that can be run and managed with certainty. The problem is that the body is not a machine. Even when we remove as much uncertainty from pregnancy and birth as possible, say with an elective scheduled cesarean, we still cannot create certainty for the process, the recovery, or the parenthood that follows. By believing in the illusion of control, we miss the opportunity to embrace some of the great teachings offered by birth: opening to the unexpected and developing greater resilience.

Pregnancy and childbirth resist methods of control. Not that we haven't tried! Whether we look at the efforts of the 1950s twilight sleep era, the more recent trend toward scheduled cesareans for calendar management, or labor inductions, methods intended to control are pervasive in birth. Over the past twenty years, I have watched as the desire to control the unpredictable nature of birth has grown. One pronounced trend is the increase in both scheduled cesareans and labor inductions. A recent survey found that "over half (53%) of all mothers experienced medical and/or self-attempts to induce labor."[2]

Reasons for Inducing Labor

The reasons mothers gave for labor induction in the report, *Listening to Mothers III* by the organization Childbirth Connection included the following:
- Baby was at full term (44%)
- Mother wanted pregnancy to be over (19%)
- Mother wanted control over timing of the birth (11%)
- Mother wanted to give birth with a specific provider (10%)

From the doctor's perspective, the reasons for induction were:
- Mother was overdue (the majority gave birth at 39.9 weeks) (18%)
- Size of the baby (16%)[3]

Control is not solely the province of modern medicine; the natural birth movement has its own ways of attempting to control birth. In the natural birth realms, the battle over control often pits pregnant people against medicine. The argument espouses that if you are smart enough to educate yourself, to increase your knowledge about birth and arm yourself for the battle of parent versus doctor, you will be able to control the outcome of your childbirth experience. While knowledge and preparation can and do help, they still cannot control the unpredictable aspects of birth. The modes of control in the natural birth model are perhaps less obvious as they often masquerade as affirmations, but the ideal is no less systemic.

The leading cry for control in the natural birth communities revolves around the need for information. It is possible to know a lot about birth, especially the physiological and technological aspects—the knowledge-based aspects of birth. But all the information and experience in the world cannot account for the uncontrollable and unknowable parts of birth, like environmental factors and emotional and spiritual experiences, as well as the actions and behaviors of others, including the baby. This is equally true of parenthood and life!

Even those with years of experience in childbirth cannot plan or control the process of their own labor experience. Loss of control is inherent in both birth and parenthood. The birthing experience of Becca, a fellow birth professional, colleague, and friend is an example of this. Becca was an experienced doula when she gave birth for the first time. Her son was her ninety-ninth birth. Armed with lots of professional know-how and understanding, Becca planned for a home birth with an obstetrician, midwife, and doula. And yet, even with all of her hard-earned wisdom as a birth professional and the expertise of her team, control was still not possible. Becca's birth had something else in store for her. She gave birth at a hospital aided by a vacuum extraction.

This was several years ago, and Becca has done a lot of healing since then. She now describes the birth as a learning experience that made her more humble and helped her to shed expectations about what a "good" (or "bad") birth means. It was also a calling to do some deep personal work around some past trauma that, following her son's birth, she discovered she needed. Birth can do that sometimes—bring psychological and emotional issues to the surface where they can be worked with or learned from. Additionally, Becca's experience has impacted her work with pregnant parents, shifting the focus from achieving some idealized birth outcome to helping them build tools that support resilience.

An openness to the unbidden and strong resilience are needed in parenthood too. Developing those skills now for labor, birth, and postpartum will support you in your long role as a parent. Let's explore some of the modes for attempting to establish control and certainty over childbirth and what you can do instead to practice opening to the unbidden and building resilience.

MODES FOR CREATING AN ILLUSION OF CONTROL AND CERTAINTY IN CHILDBIRTH

Let's look at two common modes for creating an illusion of control in birth: due dates and birth plans.

Due Dates

In pregnancy, the illusion of precision and predictability begins almost immediately after conception. If you're pregnant, you know your due date. If anyone close to you still has paper calendars (in-laws for example) your due date is likely starred and highlighted with colors and sunbursts noting it as the auspicious day that "baby" will arrive!

When I was newly pregnant with my first son, I did what so many excited soon-to-be parents do: I took not one, but two at-home pregnancy tests. Both came back positive. Since I was about to leave on a trip to Asia with my sister, I wanted to be sure before I left that I was indeed pregnant, as being pregnant would change how I might eat, drink, and care for myself while away. At my doctor's office on the

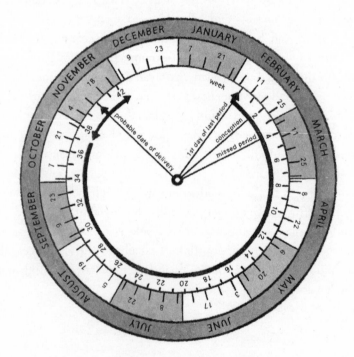

way to the airport, I took yet another pregnancy test, but this one was negative. My doctor told me this test was likely right and those taken at home false positives. Technology in the hands of the medical model was the arbiter of truth.

But I knew I was pregnant in that way that pregnant people often do. I asked if there was a more accurate test we could do to confirm my pregnancy. Ultimately, I had my blood drawn for such a test and called my husband from Laos a few days later for the "confirmation." Once confirmed by this test, my pregnancy, as determined by the medical team, officially began and its expected end was also established in terms of a due date. In our case that date was April 15, tax day, a fitting date for my husband, who is a Certified Financial Planner.

The due date is often determined by a due date calculating wheel (see image). To use this paper tool, you move the inner circle so that an arrow points at the first day of your last menstrual period. The large arrow at forty weeks points at the due date, labeled on the wheel I have as "probable date of delivery." *Probable date of delivery*!? Statements like that one start parents off believing in a sense of predictability and certainty where in fact there is very little of either.

Nowadays, you can sign up for emails tracking your baby's development week-by-week through online sites, follow your pregnancy progression through apps, and count down the number of weeks and days left until your baby arrives, all according to your due date. The attachment to this particular date is ever growing, but the actual number of babies born on their exact due date is extremely low—only about 5 percent.[5] According to research done by Rebecca Dekker of Evidence Based Birth, "Half of pregnant people go into labor naturally by 40 weeks and 5 days, and the other half go longer. Most people (90%) will go into labor on their own by 42 weeks."[6] Breaking that down, for first-time parents nearly half of all labors only spontaneously begin after forty weeks and six days! Half of all labors begin at least six days "*late*!"

While the due date is a central focus in pregnancy, it is, at least for most parents, a false target upon which to attach one's hopes. But even with the possibility of fluctuation and the variation in accuracy, due dates are held as pregnancy gospel.

Statistics Can Be Deceiving

In their book, *The Numbers Game*, journalist Michael Blastland and economist Andrew Dilnot address the changing length of pregnancy:

> Two facts about pregnancy suggest that the simple average will be misleading. First, some mothers give birth prematurely. Second, almost no one is allowed to go more than two weeks beyond the due date before being induced. Premature births pull the average down; late ones would push it up, but we physically intervene to stop babies being more than two weeks late. The effect of this imbalance—we count very early births but prevent the very late ones—is to produce a lower average than if nature were left to its own devices.[4]

The reduction in the average length of pregnancy has been artificially altered and has shortened our general perception of what is normal.

Having a sense of when your baby will come is helpful. Armed with this information, parents can plan for leave from work and arrange family travel, and medical support teams can plan their workload. Having a sense of the *approximate* time a baby will arrive is not the problem. The real challenge is the adherence to a *specific date* and the belief that that date *means something predictable*.

Another Approach

My purpose in writing this book and working with parents in the way I do is to help expand expectations of what is possible *and* how expanding expectations can help you better prepare for birth and new parenthood. Rather than adhere to the idea that your baby will arrive on a certain date, try expanding your expectations by translating your due date into a due *range*. Remember that the normal gestation period for full-term births ranges from thirty-seven weeks to forty-two weeks. That's a five-week window, not a single day on the calendar!

When asked when your baby is due, give a range instead of a single due date. For example, my due date with my first son was April 15.

		SEPTEMBER				
sun	mon	tues	weds	thurs	fri	sat
		1	2	3	4	5
6	7	8	9	10 *38 weeks*	11	12
13	14	15	16	17 *39 weeks*	18	19
20	21	22	23	24 *DUE DATE!*	25	26
27	28	29	30			

		OCTOBER				
sun	mon	tues	weds	thurs	fri	sat
				1 *41 weeks*	2	3
4	5	6	7	8 *42 weeks*	9	10
11	12	13	14	15	16	17
18	19	20	21	22	23	24
25	26	27	28	29	30	31

This is an easy one for answering with a range. I could simply answer, "April," since that covered the four-week window during which he was most likely to be born. It can be more challenging to determine a likely range when the due date falls less centrally in a month.

Let's take a due date of September 24 as another example (see figure). This date could be translated into a due range by going two to three weeks prior to the due date and two weeks after, making the answer to when are you due sound something like, "sometime in September or early October" or even looser, "sometime this fall." Kensington Palace announced Meghan Markle and Prince Harry's baby as due in the "spring" rather than giving the public a specific due date.[7]

Practicing answering in this way helps *you* begin to think about the probable time frame for birth in more expanded terms. In so doing, if you give birth earlier than your due date, you may feel less surprised. And perhaps even more important, especially if you are a first-time parent, is the expansion of the due range *beyond* the due date. I have known many parents who shared their due date with family and friends and then felt like a watched pot in the days after their due date passed when the questions started: "Are you still pregnant?" "Shouldn't you have had your baby by now?" Or, "Are you sure you shouldn't go to the hospital?"

Parents can feel like they've been pregnant forever, and they often fixate upon the due date as their likely time of salvation. Expanding the due range to include the weeks after the due date can help soften the feelings of "being late." The idea of being "late" implies that being "on time" means giving birth on a single date rather than sometime during a rather large-sized chunk of dates on the calendar.

The Birth Plan

Writing a birth plan has become a standard part of the preparatory journey for most birthing parents. There is no shortage of recommendations on writing birth plans—outlines and suggested formats are available online and in almost every book on childbirth.

Plans are designs intended to control events—they give the impression of inevitability. Merriam-Webster's primary definition of *plan* is "a set of actions that have been thought of as a way to do or achieve something."[8] To write a birth plan is to design a way to achieve a specific outcome, which in turn and more damagingly, creates greater attachment to that outcome.

Writing a birth plan can give parents a false sense of control over how birth will unfold, as if doing this seemingly obligatory prenatal homework and writing a thorough-enough birth plan can control the events of birth.

Some research has shown that the differences in outcome between those with a birth plan and those without are marginal at best.[9] It is horrifying to me that 65 percent of doctors *believe* that those patients with birth plans are more likely to have a cesarean or have worse outcomes even though the rates of cesarean and episiotomy are about equal between those with and without a birth plan.[10]

Here's part of the problem: Birth plans are often presented to medical staff at birth and stand as the primary mode of communication between parents and their provider regarding desires and wishes for birth. But this is often too late in the process. Not all birth options are available with every health-care provider or in every birth setting. Unless your provider (and their team), as well as your intended birth setting, are supportive of the options you learn about, birth plans can prove futile in creating specific birth outcomes. It is rare to get care that is different from what is usually offered by individual care providers in their usual care settings.[11]

Not that birth plans are a complete waste of time or always a negative. The *practice* of writing a birth plan can be very helpful in educating parents about the possibilities that can occur in birth and work as a great launching pad for insightful conversations with your provider *prenatally*. But if instead the act of writing a birth plan concretizes your ideas about how birth will go, it can add to the illusion of control and work against you.

A Different Plan for Birth Plans

What's the alternative? Writing a birth plan as a *process* in your overall education can help inform you about commonplace procedures in labor, birth, and early postpartum. This process of self-education is a good exercise.

If you feel inspired to write out your preferences, use your preference sheet as a tool for communication with your care provider *well in advance* of labor. I recommend exploring the options for labor, birth, and postpartum as early in pregnancy as possible because you might discover that your intentions for birth conflict with the routine practices of your provider. Such an incongruent relationship may necessitate an unexpected change in your hired support. While changing care providers is usually possible throughout pregnancy, it's often easier to do earlier rather than later.

Think of a birth plan as a tool for educating yourself and communicating with your care provider so that you can learn how compatible your preferences are with those typically available with your selected medical team and birth location. Birth plans get trickiest when they lay out your preferences like a script for labor that should be followed by all actors. There are too many actors involved and too many external and internal factors in labor and birth to be able to predict whether your birth will follow the script. Basically, labor doesn't read scripts.

Birth Intentions

Try going beyond a birth plan by writing out your *intentions* instead. Intentions are very different from goals. Goals are measurable and therefore can either succeed or fail, whereas intentions address *how* you would like to be with yourself and others. Here's an example:

- Goal: to birth without drugs

- Intention: to labor strongly, with focus and attention to what is needed in the moment, to ask for help when I need it, and to be tender with myself even when I don't feel powerful

These feel different both now and in labor: one sets us up to either succeed or fail, while the other prepares us to be strong, focused, and gentle with ourselves in each moment, regardless of the path the labor takes.

So what are your intentions for labor and birth? Here are some prompts you might want to consider:

- How do you intend to be with yourself in moments of intensity or struggle?

- How do you intend to be with yourself in moments of great joy?

- How do you intend to be with your partner? Labor support? Care providers?

- How do you intend to be with the ever-changing nature of birth?

- If you find yourself losing track of your intentions, how would you like to be supported in coming back to focus?

- If things go in ways other than you desire, how do you wish to be with those unwished-for changes?

Be wary of answering these questions in order to please others, or as a means of getting the birth outcome you most desire. It may be helpful to think about things *not* going exactly the way you most hope they do and answering from within that scenario. You don't have to focus too much here on action plans for how'll you'll be if things don't go as you imagine. In chapter 8 we will explore strategies for building greater resilience and how to work with your concerns about labor, birth, and postpartum.

Writing out intentions for birth can look more like writing a guided meditation for yourself, one that reminds you what is truly important about how you wish to show up for yourself, your partner, and your baby in all the ways labor and birth might unfold.

Here are some examples of birth intentions:

- I intend to follow my body's desire for movement, water, food, temperature, light or darkness, sound, and vocalization—knowing my preferences may fluctuate and change over time.

- I intend to practice receiving help from those around me when needed.

- I intend to let myself refuse help when it does not suit me in the moment.

- I intend to remember I am not alone, that I am working with my baby.

- I intend to connect with the love around me and the love I feel for my baby.

- I intend to make decisions about my care in the moment when the conversation arises and ask for help in getting the information I need to make choices that feel appropriate for me at the time.

- I intend to give myself permission to be impolite and antisocial if that is what I need.

- I intend to be kind with myself if things surprise me, and I find those surprises difficult.

- I intend to make myself large enough to feel all the emotions that need to be felt, even those I find difficult or unsavory in my prelabor state.

These are just a few possibilities. What are your intentions? How do you want to hold yourself through the experience of labor and birth? Try writing them out. Keep them to a single page, and keep them simple, if possible. Once you have them down, work with them. Read them often. Use them as guiding principles for your life leading up to labor. I like to think of birth intentions like wedding vows. They guide your actions from a place of profound love and commitment. This time, the love and commitment are to yourself, your baby, and perhaps, your partner. If you prefer, you can write them as, "To the best of my ability, I will . . ." Use what works for you!

If, after writing down your intentions, you still feel compelled to write a traditional birth plan, follow these suggestions:

- Write it early and use it as a tool for dialoguing with your medical team at prenatal appointments.

- Keep it to under one page in length.

- Address only those aspects most important to you.

- Ask birth professionals in your area (specifically doulas and childbirth educators) how birth plans are received at the birth setting you plan to use.

- Most importantly, hold it with flexibility and an openness to the unbidden.

As addressed in this chapter, you can't know how your birth will unfold; certainty is an illusion. No birth plan, no matter how many pages long, could possibly address every unknown and unique possibility for your labor. And, you still need to be able to get the information you need to make the best possible decisions and advocate for your desires and rights in labor. I will discuss how to do this in chapter 8.

4

Too Much Information!

How often have you been sitting for a meal with friends or family and someone says, "I wonder . . . ?" only to have someone instantly pick up their smartphone to Google the answer? It happens so often that I've nicknamed my iPhone the "Wonder Killer," as we rarely sit in wonder, captivated by curiosity as we discuss the possible answers to the question.

THE VENERATION OF INFORMATION AND TECHNOLOGY

We live in a world where information is readily available. The idea that parents need more information for labor and birth stems in part from our strong belief in science—science is a reigning god in our cultural mythology.

If information were all it took to have a particular type of birth experience or to parent exceptionally well, we would have a world full of amazing births and phenomenally raised children. This is simply not the case. Thriving during birth and parenthood requires so much more than intellectually knowing information.

For many parents on the journey into birth and parenthood, childbirth classes are an essential part of arming themselves for birth. Sadly, these courses are often focused entirely on educating and imparting *information* to new parents. Charts, graphs, and slide presentations are now relatively commonplace in childbirth education classes. Heads are filled with facts and figures, even though bodies do the work of labor. When I took classes in preparation for the birth of my first child in 2000, I sought out alternative classes. Even though I looked for something more all-encompassing, the classes I attended were almost exclusively informational—imparting data and statistics about labor and birth. There was very little focus on *preparation* for birth beyond adding information on the topic.

Understanding the cultural addiction to information doesn't mean we should abandon all efforts to gain knowledge about important topics. Information is powerful, to a point. In addition to gaining intellectual understanding, we must also transmute that information into embodied wisdom that is both accessible and useable when needed. Disembodied information acts to further separate us from our bodies and our animal nature. We are not machines where inputting data in the form of charts and graphs yields standard results.

Information without reflection or practice does little to support the transformative experience of birth. Addiction to the promise of information only puts us at a greater disadvantage in early parenthood when few concrete answers exist. We must revalue curiosity, embodied practice, and wonder.

RECONNECT WITH WONDER

We have lost our ability to sit in wonder, to hold the discomfort associated with not knowing. It is too easy to get immediate answers to any question. Information is *always* available. With easy access to "answers," we spend less time hanging out with uncertainty and ambiguity. We have become wary of wonder and its partner, curiosity. When we feel these, we believe there is an answer that we are simply missing. While seeking an answer is fundamental to human nature, something has changed in this Information Age. What's different is the way we handle wonder and curiosity now that we live with constant access to the internet and its unlimited answers. The speed at which we reach out for an answer causes us to lose connection with our intuition and reduces our belief in our own ability to come to an answer all on our own. This ability has been replaced by a belief that a *right* answer exists out there.

In my classes, I am frequently asked, "How long are contractions?" "How long is too long for water to be broken before a baby is born?" "Should I do delayed cord clamping?" "Is it better to encapsulate my placenta or do cord blood banking?" These questions are asked as if there is a right answer that is universally true for everyone. Guess what? There are no universal answers to any of these.

So, what's a parent to do on the quest for information to ensure that they have the best transition through birth and into parenthood? The first step is to expand the pause. It is in the space between question and answer where you can take the time to inquire within, to ponder an answer, to explore your feelings, and to ask yourself what you need to know. It is within that place where we become reacquainted with wonder.

The next step is to ask *yourself*. Once you've expanded the pause between the question and the knee-jerk reaction to find an answer, go a little deeper within yourself. Ask yourself what you need to know and what you *already* know. Then inquire within yourself about how best to get the information you need. Would the internet, doctor, friend, family member, book, or podcast be your best option to help you explore this further? Practice and hone this skill in pregnancy as it is a crucial skill in parenting.

The third step is to explore the ranges. Once you've expanded the pause and asked yourself about what you already know and inquired how to best get the missing knowledge, then explore the ranges. Rather than seeking singular answers to questions, investigate what is possible. Let's take length of contractions as an example. Contractions have a range of normal. Some are only a few seconds while others can last a couple of minutes. Then there is the perceived experience of contractions that go beyond clock time. Asking how long contractions are implies that clock time makes sense in labor. Some contractions are short and yet feel like they go on forever, while others are long and yet can be totally managed. Rather than looking for a definitive answer to how long contractions last, ask yourself how you will keep going regardless of how long a contraction *feels*. That's what matters.

Similarly, couples often ask me how long postpartum lasts as if there were a marker that could be placed on a calendar that would signify when postpartum ends. Even though modern medical practice has a post-birth six-week postpartum checkup, this in no way should suggest that the postpartum experience is complete by that time. Alternatively, it is also sometimes stated that postpartum lasts a year, even though some parents report still feeling deep in postpartum long after their child's first birthday. Concrete time markers say almost nothing about the *inner* experience had by the individual. Concrete markers work well in books, not births.

Try This

Going Within

The next time you have a moment of "I wonder," practice these four steps:

1. Expand the pause.

2. Ask yourself how you *feel* about this topic, what you *already know* about it, what *you still need to know*, and how best to fill in any missing knowledge.

3. Look for the ranges of possibility rather than a single answer.

4. Ask yourself if there is anything else you need to know about this topic. If so, start again at number one.

Resist the temptation to follow every thread down internet rabbit holes looking for answers. Before you go looking for answers in books or online, first go within and practice these four steps. Practice giving value to the knowledge that can only be found within yourself.

THE LABYRINTH

On the path toward birth and new parenthood, of course you want to know what might support you through the journey. That's to be expected. Information has value, but we must remember that it is only one part, and expanding our ability to face the unknowable aspects of birth and parenthood is critical. One of my favorite metaphors for the journey of giving birth and becoming a parent that aids in understanding intellectually *and* expands your capacity to hold wonder is the labyrinth. (I am forever grateful to my teacher, Pam England, for lighting a fire within me for this simple and yet profound symbol.)

Labyrinths are often confused with mazes. Mazes are made with the intention to confuse, disorient, and ideally, get you lost. But labyrinths are different. Unlike mazes, labyrinths are designed for contemplation, prayer, ritual, and meditation. The most basic form of labyrinth is a simple spiral, which has one opening that serves as both entrance and exit and a single path that leads to the center. Labyrinths, from simple spirals to complex twisting patterns, are found all over the world carved into stones, built into the ground, made from rocks, planted as hedges, drawn into the sand, crafted in mosaics and stone on the floors of buildings, and pictured on antique coins. They show up in folklore, myths, and legends (I'll share a Greek labyrinth myth later).

Understanding the powerful symbolic nature of labyrinths is best explored through drawing, tracing, and/or walking one. Since I can't know where you are as you read this, or if there is a labyrinth near you to walk, I'll instruct you on drawing a basic labyrinth. If you are reading this book with your partner, I invite you to each make your own.

Try This

Drawing a Labyrinth

You'll need a piece of paper, preferably a large piece somewhere from 12 x 16 to 22 x 30. Any paper will do, even a sheet of printer paper will work, but it's best if it doesn't have lines. You'll also need something to draw with. I like chalk pastels or paint best as they're more unpredictable like birth, but colored pencils, crayons, or markers are also fine, especially if that's all you have.

To draw the labyrinth, you'll need to start by "planting" the seed pattern from which your labyrinth will grow. If your paper is a rectangle, turn the paper sideways so that it's wider than it is tall. From left to right, find the center of your paper. Then, find the spot that is one third up from the bottom and two thirds down from the top of the paper and place a plus sign. Next, you'll draw the corner lines, which are right angles that mirror the shape of the inside of each of the angles of the plus sign. Allow enough room for your finger to fit between the plus sign lines and your new right-angle lines.

The last step in making the seed pattern is to place a dot up from each of the right-angle corners. Once you have made the plus sign, the right-angle lines and the four dots, your seed pattern is done (see figure to the right).

Now, grow the labyrinth from the seed and make the pathways. Start at the top of the vertical line of your plus sign and from there draw an upside-down U that connects the top of that line to the first line on the right (see the figure below). This is the center of your labyrinth and for our metaphoric purposes, is the place your baby is born.

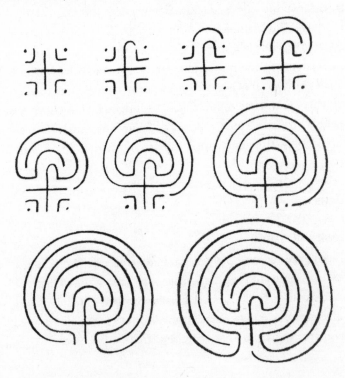

Next find the first line to the left of the center line and draw a line from the top of it, up and over the previous line you drew to the dot to the right of the last spot you connected making a pathway-like space between the first line and this new line. Go back to the *left*. This time, you'll connect the dot on the *left* up and over to the next available line on the *right*. Keep going from the left up and over to the right, connecting the next line or dot on the *left* to the next line or dot on the *right*, always going up and over, until all lines and all dots have been connected to another one and there is only one entrance/exit at the bottom of the labyrinth.

Add a threshold stone near the entrance. Some labyrinths have these, others do not. The threshold stone is a reminder to pause and mark the separation from outside to inside the labyrinth. Thresholds are meant to be places that mark transitions *and* draw attention to that transition. Threshold stones are helpful for our purpose, so go ahead and draw one just in front of the entrance. It can be as simple or as creatively elaborate as you like. Your labyrinth should resemble the image here.

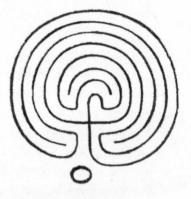

Now that you have a completed labyrinth, place your fingers near the entrance in front of the threshold. This is where you are now in relation to your birth. All of what you know about *your* birth experience is outside of the labyrinth. When labor starts, you step over the threshold stone and enter the journey that is uniquely yours. Take your fingers and follow the pathway—the space between the lines—to the center of the labyrinth. Pause in the center and reflect on the following:

- What did you notice? How might what you noticed be like birth?

- What surprised you? How might that be like birth?

- What was it like to come to the right-angle turns? What about the U-turns that seem to take you away from the center? What are potential U-turns in labor or birth?

- When tracing a labyrinth pathway with a finger after drawing it, it's normal to think you have drawn it wrong or made some sort of mistake, since the turns seem to take you farther away from the center rather than closer. How might that experience be similar to birth?

- At any point did you think you had made a wrong turn or skipped a line? How might that be like labor or birth?

- There are no dead ends or wrong turns in labyrinths like there are in mazes. What did it take to get to the center? You have to keep going and stay mindful of where you are . . . just like in labor.

Everything inside the labyrinth is your labor. Everything outside the labyrinth is what you know about your labor journey beforehand, all that you know about birth in general, and who you are today. You're waiting, paused at the entrance, not sure when you will step across the threshold and enter. Will your water break first, like is so often the case in movies . . . a giant gush all at once, in a very public place, and the need to run fast, screaming, to the nearest hospital because your baby will be born in mere minutes? Only about one in ten labors start with the water breaking or a rupture of the membranes as it is also called (FYI: PROM stands for premature rupture of membranes and AROM stands for artificial rupture of membranes, which in laypeople's language is known as breaking the water).[1]

So how do the other nine out ten labors begin? How do most people know when their labor starts? This can be tricky to determine. Many people have contractions well before labor begins. Maybe you're already having some of those contractions known widely as Braxton Hicks contractions—named after Dr. John Braxton Hicks who in 1872 "identified" them.[2] Since I am quite sure pregnant people long before 1872 had been experiencing this type of contraction, I prefer to refer to these as "practice" or "warm-up" contractions. For first-time parents, determining the difference between warm-up contractions and the real deal can be hard. I like to suggest what a midwife once told me that she recommends her clients do: if you're having contractions, drink a big glass of water (dehydration can stimulate practice contractions) and change positions (meaning if you're lying down, get up and if you've been active, lie down and rest). If the contractions stop, you likely aren't in labor. If they stick around and intensify, it could be the start of labor.

If this sounds vague, that's because it is. Often parents spend time wondering whether or not they have stepped across the threshold into their labor. It's almost like doing the cha-cha over the threshold stone of the labyrinth: "Yay! I'm in labor! Oh, wait, maybe not . . ." in and out, never sure if it's really happening or not. Usually, at some point, the contractions intensify, lengthen, and often become regular. Keep going on with your life until you can't do otherwise. When you are *unable* to do anything except focus on the contractions, then you're likely in labor. We'll discuss more about how labor progresses a bit later.

Sometimes, parents enter the labyrinth of birth with a conversation with their health-care provider about scheduling an induction or a cesarean. There are no shortcuts through the labyrinth. These sorts of conversations are another way to step over the threshold stone and enter the labyrinth of birth.

The labyrinth, like the experience of giving birth, twists and turns as the path makes its way toward the center. Not every path *feels* like it's taking you closer, even if it ultimately does. Some turns take you in the opposite direction of where you intend to go—turning toward the exit on your way to the center or toward the center on your way toward the exit. Walking or tracing a labyrinthine path often leaves you confused or disoriented. Even if the path has no wrong turns, it can still feel like you've done something wrong as you traverse it. The only thing you have to do to make it to the center of a labyrinth is to intentionally stay on the path and *keep going*. That's it. The path will guide you toward the center. The same is true in labor: to make your way to birth you have to practice staying in the moment, taking only one step at a time, and keep going.

We're going to leave labyrinths for now, although I will refer to them regularly throughout the book as they are foundational to how I discuss labor, birth, and postpartum. Remember that you traced your way to the center of the labyrinth, but you haven't come out yet. We'll do that later when we explore postpartum.

THE LANGUAGE OF BIRTH

There are very few concrete truths in birth and few reliable mile markers along the way through labor. This makes discussing how labor works difficult; hence the labyrinth. Most attempts to explain how labor works give the impression that there is a single linear way birth progresses, and that birth unfolds exactly as it is laid out in books . . . in *books*! Labor doesn't read the books that tell it how to progress. Still, there are some things that are helpful to understand. One of them is the language and terminology of birth.

Imagine you are heading to a country you've never been to before. Its landscape, people, and language are all unfamiliar to you. In preparation for your trip, you get a few guide books, do some research, learn a few helpful phrases in the language spoken in that country, and maybe even hire a guide or translator to help you while you're there. Labor is a lot like going to a country you've never been to. It's unfamiliar, and they speak a different language. All of the preparatory endeavors you would engage in to travel to a truly unknown country you need to do in preparation for birth. Let's start with a language lesson.

Physiology

In the simplest of terms, labor is the process of opening the body enough for the baby to exit. Opening is the main activity of birth. But your body isn't the only thing that needs to open. Many things need to open. Your mind has to open to unexpected events. Your comfort level has to open and expand to accept the ways you may behave or sound during labor. Your relationships and family have to open to welcome a new member. Your lifestyle has to open to accommodate the needs of a dependent newborn. Your identity has to open to the role of parent. And your heart has to open wide and expand to hold the love. Modern birth culture, however, is fixated on one type of opening: dilation.

Dilation

The cervix (the entrance to the uterus) has to open in order for the baby to be born. The uterus actually pulls back to open rather than gradually enlarging like a shutter on a camera lens. Imagine putting on a turtleneck shirt with a tight opening. As you pull the turtleneck down over your head it expands and opens to allow your head to come through the opening. This is not entirely unlike what your baby's head does with the cervix. Do you see the thick "turtleneck-like" bulge under the baby's head and above the vagina in the figure here? That's the cervix.

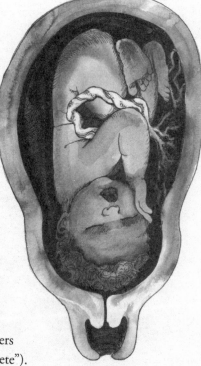

The process of opening the cervix is called *dilation*. This is the most common word in labor language because of our cultural fixation on progress, which many believe can be gauged by the amount of dilation. Dilation is measured in centimeters from zero (or closed) to ten (or "complete").

Measuring the dilation in quantifiable terms makes it *seem* like dilation is an objective and stable measurement that can be relied upon. Isn't that what numbers are for—to make things quantifiable and reliable?

Here's the thing. We have to consider *how* this measurement is taken. There isn't a mechanized caliper that is inserted into the vagina that expands, beeps, and comes out with a "factual measurement" (not that I wish there were!). Cervical dilation is measured by a medical professional (nurse, midwife, or doctor) performing a vaginal exam. To do this, they insert their fingers into the vagina and use them to determine the amount of dilation from zero to ten centimeters (see the figure below). For whatever reason, while they do this, it seems as if the answer they are looking for is on the ceiling as they usually look there! Is this an objective foolproof process of measurement? Far from it. While health-care providers specializing in birth are well trained and have performed this procedure often, likely thousands of times, it is still prone to differences based on unreliable variables such as hand size, experience, location of the cervix in relation to the pelvis, ease of the check, whether the check was done during a contraction or not, and good old human error. It is a subjective measurement that seems to rule our culture's understanding of labor progress!

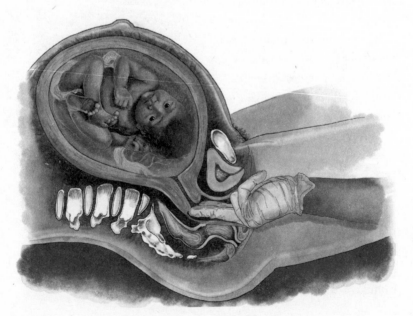

Effacement

In addition to opening, the cervix also has to thin. The process of thinning is called *effacement* and is shown in the figure below. Remember our turtleneck example before? Think of the whole neck of the turtleneck as representing the thick bulbous cervix prior to labor. As the turtleneck pulls back over the head, the thickness of the neck (cervix) decreases even before the opening expands. This is like cervical effacement, which is measured in percentages and ranges from 0 percent effaced (completely thick and bulbous) to 100 percent effaced (completely thinned out to what is sometimes referred to as "paper thin"). As with dilation, this measurement is subjective in nature, leaving a lot of room for practitioner interpretation.

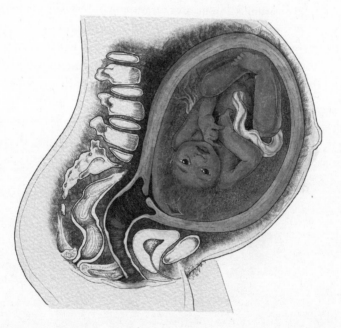

What can be helpful to know about effacement, especially for first-time birthing parents, is that it's common for effacement to happen almost completely *before* dilation makes much progress. That means that while you might be laboring for hours and making little to no progress in dilation, something else important is likely still happening. Just because ours is a dilation-focused birth culture doesn't mean that dilation is the only measurement of progress.

Position of Baby

In terms of the language of birth, there are a few ways that the position and location of the baby are addressed. Commonly, medical providers tell parents only two things: whether baby is positioned head up or head down and whether baby is *floating* or *engaged* in the pelvis. Sometimes rather than saying floating or engaged, they simply refer to high or low. Floating, or high, is when the baby's presenting part (usually the head) is not yet locked in to the pelvic bowl and can be more easily moved around within the abdomen. Engaged, or low, refers to when the presenting feature is locked in to the pelvis and the baby is more settled into its position. While somewhat helpful, these pieces of information are very limited. And, as with measuring dilation and effacement, position is a subjective measurement made by the provider based on experience, training, and hands-on palpitation.

Providers may pronounce to one another (but not usually to the parents) the *station* of the baby. This term refers to where the presenting part of the baby is in relation to the ischial spines of the parent's pelvis (as shown in the figure below). Providers differ in which scale they use either -5 to +5 or -3 to +3 but all have zero at the place where the baby's head is aligned with the ischial spines and engaged in the pelvis.

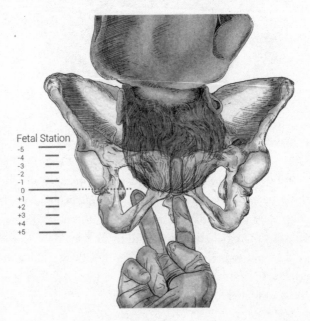

Fetal Station
-5
-4
-3
-2
-1
0
+1
+2
+3
+4
+5

The negative numbers indicate where the head is higher in the pelvis or abdomen. Negative four or five would be considered floating and the baby's presenting part is palpable outside of the pelvic area. Babies are usually born at +4 or +5, which is the point where the baby has descended not just into the pelvis, but moved under the pubic bone, through the birth canal, and all the way to the vaginal opening.

In class when I demonstrate stations with a model pelvis and parents see baby at zero, it can look like there's not much left as the opening of the pelvis is right by the baby's head. Then, I strap the cloth vagina onto the model pelvis and everything changes! After zero, the baby still needs to tuck under the pubic bone and move through the birth canal. The baby can, and often does, bulge the vaginal opening. Even if the top of the baby's head has moved mostly through the pelvic opening, it still has a distance to travel through the soft tissue. These are the positive numbers that go all the way to +5 . . . although at that point, few people are talking about stations as they're now discussing birth!

The station is one aspect of positioning. Another less common, but highly important part of fetal positioning has to do with which way the baby is facing—front or back, or left or right. An anterior position is where the baby's back is facing toward the front of the parent's belly. A posterior position is where the baby's back is facing toward the parent's spine, as it is in the figure shown here.

Right and left is determined by where the back of the baby's head (or occiput) is in relation to the parent's body. If the parent feels kicks on the right side, the baby is likely positioned on the left, and if the parent feels the kicks on the left, the baby is likely positioned on the right. While labors can work with several different fetal positions, they tend to be quicker and sometimes easier when baby is on the left and anterior. While this is more than some medical providers usually discuss with parents, I've only shared a small fraction of what can be helpful to know about optimal fetal positioning for labor. If this is interesting to you and you'd like to help baby get into a good position for labor, I highly recommend learning more from the Spinning Babies website or a Spinning Babies instructor in your area.

Stages of Labor

We've discussed some of the medical terms used to express progress in labor: dilation, effacement, and stations. *Stages* is another term in labor that can be vague and confusing, as it is understood in various ways by different people.

According to medical terminology the three stages of labor are as follows:

- First stage: the period from the start of labor to the complete dilation of the cervix (see figure)

- Second stage: the period from complete dilation to birth of the baby (sometimes referred to as the "pushing stage")

- Third stage: the birth of the placenta

For most parents the phrase "stages of labor" refers to the three phases that occur *within* the first stage and are called *early*, *active*, and *transition*. These are often the terms parents use when telling their birth stories.

In my years of teaching, the definitions of early, active, and transition have changed. This is both interesting and important to know because

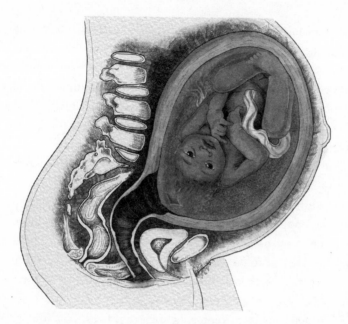

once something has a name and a definition, we think it is set, solid, and unchanging. While we crave clear classifications in birth—and in life—few exist. Even definitions are fluid and changeable! While the term *stages* makes it seem like there are levels of progression that are clear and definable, this is not really the case either. And even when a labor seems to follow the stages, it still doesn't mean much about what will happen next, as every minute is an opportunity for labor to chart its own unique course. Keeping in mind the fluid nature of these terms, let's explore them further.

In terms of definition, early labor is referred to as the time from when labor begins until the cervix has dilated to five centimeters. When I started teaching, early labor was until three centimeters or four centimeters! That's a big difference in only two decades. But since you likely won't know how dilated your cervix is without a cervical check, the definition might not be very helpful. What might be more helpful is to understand how early labor behaves.

Early labor is that period of time when labor is figuring itself out. I sometimes describe it as being like a train leaving the station: it takes a while for the wheels of labor to really start rolling. Early labor is usually the least uniform of all the stages and is where labor is most likely to be negatively affected by outside influences. It might start and stop; some contractions might be fifteen seconds long while others are ninety. Contractions might be regular with a consistent amount of time between them ranging from five to ten minutes, or the time between them might vary—five minutes apart, then ten, then three, then eight, and so on. Early labor might have a pattern, or it might seem random. It can last for a few hours or a few days.

One of the hardest parts about early labor is that it rarely feels early to a first-time parent, because it's the first experience of labor the parent has ever had! Early labor may feel *hard* and it likely is, and while the body is doing important work, there is still lots more to do. It's common for parents in early labor to think they are further along than they are and to face disappointment when upon a cervical exam they learn they are hardly dilated at all or only at two or three centimeters and may be sent home to labor further before being admitted to the hospital or birth center. In such moments, it is important to remember the labyrinth—labor is not a linear process and dilation is only one of the medical measurements for progress.

One of the leading causes of unnecessary medical interventions in labor is something called "failure to progress." This is the phrase used when labor doesn't progress according to medical expectations. Progress in early labor does not follow a predictable, clear, linear, sloping line. As such, labeling a labor as a "failure to progress" while still in early labor often leads to unnecessary interventions including cesareans. In 2014, the American College of Obstetrics and Gynecology (ACOG) presented a consensus paper to its community in an effort to safely reduce the rate of primary cesareans.[4] This announcement expanded the length of early labor to include everything up to and including five centimeters. That means labor shouldn't be expected to have a strong regular pattern until after six centimeters, when active labor begins, giving the labor train more of a chance to gain momentum and truly leave the station.

Active labor is usually that time when all energy must go toward the labor itself: the mind's focus turns inward even between contractions, distractions can be highly irritating, and even talking becomes difficult. During this period, every ounce of energy is needed to help ride the waves of each contraction. Sometimes, you vomit. During active labor, contractions are usually at least a minute long and coming regularly with only a few minutes between them. Active labor is no joke. It is often hard and intense. That intensity is opening the body wide to help birth your baby.

The stage that follows active labor is transition. I've begun thinking of transition differently and as a *threshold period* woven within active labor. From my perspective, transition is characterized by the intensity of emotion that usually comes somewhere between six and ten centimeters rather than defined by a particular amount of dilation. It is that period of time when the body is opening so wide it tips the energetic flow of labor into its highest gear, and labor becomes a holding-on-by-the-fingernails experience. It is often recognizable by those moments when the parent doesn't think they can keep going . . . when tears, upset, anger, frustration, or loss of confidence are common.

Many experienced birth professionals recognize this shift as a very good sign. When parents start shedding tears and expressing great doubt in response to the immense effort and surrender labor demands, birth professionals are silently celebrating the emotional changes, as they know from experience that such expressions frequently indicate that the work of labor is truly happening and birth is coming. Often, transition feels like the train has not only left the station but is heading down the tracks so fast that everyone should just get out of its way. This period tends to be hard, emotional, and very intense. It is also the necessary threshold you often have to cross before the cervix completely opens and your baby can emerge.

While the stages of labor can help give you a sense of what is normal at different times during the process, remember the labyrinth and its twists and turns. Stages of labor imply that there is a pattern to labor, when in reality such order and predictability rarely exist. The other thing to know about stages of labor is that the person *in* labor rarely pays attention to which stage they are in. There aren't easy signs to determine one from the other. It can all feel hard. Doubt can arise anytime. Ease and flow might guide you through to birth. There are no hard and fast rules about the stages of labor and about birth in general. Your job is to stay with what's happening in the moment, rather than being in your head thinking about physiology or stages.

QUESTIONS OF TIME

One of the main questions parents want to know when they arrive at a childbirth class is how long labor will take. The desire to know how the labor and birth process will unfold is what drives many parents to childbirth classes in the first place.

In addition to the length of pregnancy being ever more narrowly defined, as I shared in the previous chapter, so too is the length of the labor itself. Every hospital labor room has a clock, and it is used not only to determine the time of the baby's birth, but, medically speaking, labor is structured and organized on principles of time. Time-based measurements are then used to map labor in terms of what is considered "normal" according to medical providers and often based on the now infamous graph known as Friedman's curve.

Friedman's curve is a graph used to explain the results of a study conducted in 1954 by Dr. Emanuel A. Friedman in which he followed the births of 500 first-time mothers. Based on his findings, he designed a graph depicting the average length of time it takes for labor to progress from one stage to another.[5] Some sixty years later, Friedman's curve is still being used and debated. In 2014 ACOG questioned Friedman's results and conducted studies with thousands of participants (as compared to Friedman's hundreds). These studies led to finding that the actual rate of dilation during the active phase is much slower than what Friedman's work suggested.[6]

Western culture loves linear progression and time as expressed on the clock. Dr. Friedman, followed by ACOG, gave Western birth culture what it so badly desires—faith in orderly progress. The focus on time in labor as arbiter of what is normal and abnormal is likely to stay.

Timing Contractions

Speaking of time, one of the most common things partners do during labor is time contractions. It makes sense—focusing on a clock, timer, or app is far more familiar and therefore more comfortable than supporting someone when they're navigating the challenges of labor. I remember the time I arrived at a client's home when she was in labor, and her husband proudly handed me a yellow pad where he had listed the length and time of every single contraction his wife had experienced thus far in labor. You don't have to do this! Timing contractions can take the focus off of what is actually happening and put the focus on a technological device instead. In the next chapter we'll discuss how focus of that sort can be detrimental to labor in general.

For people who are inexperienced with labor and what it looks like, timing contractions can be a helpful tool to use *in moderation*. There is no reason to time every contraction through the entire labor. I don't time contractions unless I want confirmation of what I already suspect is true from observation. As a tool, timing contractions is best used to determine when to go to your intended birth location if you are not already there. There's a set of numbers that can help you determine when that time has arrived, but these vary so be sure to ask your medical care provider for their recommendation. In my community, the numbers vary and I have heard 4-1-1, 5-1-1, 5-1-2, and 6-1-1. Ask your provider when they want you to call them or come to your birth location.

What do these numbers mean? The first number refers to the number of minutes between contractions. This can be deceptive because it seems like that would be the time from when a contraction ends to when the next one begins, which is not the case. The time between contractions is timed from the *start* of a contraction to the start of the next contraction as shown in the figure below. The contraction itself is included in the time between.

The second number, a 1 in the above examples, refers to the length of each contraction lasting for at least one minute. The last number

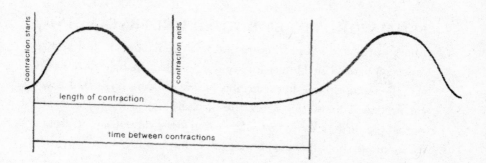

indicates how many hours this pattern should be active before going to your intended birth location. This number reminds you that you're looking for consistency and not just two contractions that last for a minute and are four minutes apart. Under normal circumstances and a healthy pregnancy, you want to aim to arrive in active labor with strong regular contractions. This number tool is intended to help inexperienced parents hit that mark. A 4-1-1 labor pattern means that contractions are four minutes apart, they're lasting for at least a minute, and this pattern has been happening for an hour. Keep in mind that means that if a contraction is a minute long, the time from the end of contraction to the start of another is only three minutes, giving parents only a short rest period before another contraction starts. This can be very intense, and many parents leave home and head for their care provider before this point because they do not want to be in the car during such an intense phase or they feel birth is imminent.

The numbers above are only a guide based on what many providers suggest in my area. There are certainly labors that move much faster or never establish a solid pattern of any sort. When in doubt, call your provider. You might be amazed by what experienced birth professionals can determine just by talking to you on the phone. Or just go . . . if you're too early, you can go back home. This happens sometimes, especially with first-time parents. One of the reasons to have a doula or someone experienced in childbirth present is to help determine when to go. While experience doesn't make the decision of "when to go" foolproof, those of us who have witnessed at least a few labors have an easier time telling how far along a labor is just by being in the space with the laboring person.

FROM WORDS TO EMBODIED UNDERSTANDING

I have just shared a lot of information with you about birth. I know expectant parents are hungry for information that can help them navigate the unknown and unpredictable nature of labor, birth, and new parenthood. I know this desire myself, and, after a few decades of working in birth, I know that information alone cannot save us from the unknown and unpredictable aspects of birth or life.

According to ethnographic photographer Jimmy Nelson, the indigenous group known as the Asaro tribe of Papua New Guinea have this proverb: "Knowledge is only rumor until it is in the muscle."[7] This saying is brilliant and so accurate in regard to birth. We can fill our minds with information, but until we have moved it into experience in the body, it doesn't count for much. So, then, what can you do to move the information from this chapter into embodied wisdom? What we most need is practice expanding our ability to navigate whatever is not planned or expected.

Try This

Letting Go of Expectations

Practice letting go when things do not go as expected. For example, let's say you are driving somewhere and there is terrible unexpected traffic (I live in Los Angeles, so this is a common occurrence that provides frequent opportunities for practice). It's nobody's fault. Traffic is just traffic. Rather than getting bent out of shape and riled up, use it as a practice of nonattachment for labor and new parenthood. Do what you need to do to tend to the unwished-for situation, such as call your appointment so they know you'll be late, change lanes or routes to facilitate the most successful navigation, and, most importantly, use your mindfulness practices, breathing exercises, or supportive self-talk to help settle into the unexpected event with as much acceptance as you can muster (but be sure to stay focused on driving). Make finding your way into being okay the highest priority. We have opportunities on a regular basis in which we can practice bringing our attention and intention to surrendering expectations rather than being tortured by rigid ideas.

Into the
Wilderness

In the previous chapter I got into some of the details about birth in terms of physiology and terminology, as well as exploring the labyrinth as a metaphor for the journey of labor. Throughout the chapter, I tried to convey the unpredictable qualities and expand expectations of normal labor and birth while simultaneously providing some basic knowledge about the process. In this chapter, I dive a bit deeper into how labor works while also continuing to explore the unknowable nature of the journey.

REVERENCE FOR ORDERED CULTURE OVER WILD NATURE

It could be said that birth has two different landscapes—the inner one experienced by those *in* labor and an outer landscape created by the culture within which labor and birth occur. Here I start to explore some mythological elements as tools to help expand and deepen your understanding of birth. In order to explain how birth works within contemporary culture, I want to introduce you to the twin Greek gods, Artemis and Apollo.

Artemis and Apollo

Artemis and Apollo, as you might remember from reading or hearing Greek myths as a child or at school, are Leto and Zeus's twins. Due to the jealous interventions of Zeus's wife Hera, Leto had a very difficult birth. Hera commanded that Leto not be given a space to birth and prevented Eileithyia, the goddess who attended women in childbirth, from helping Leto. While there are differing accounts of the births, Leto did finally give birth to Artemis. As sometimes happens in mythology, Artemis was born a full-grown goddess (imagine that labor!). Seeing her mother in distress, Artemis supported her while she gave birth to Apollo. In essence, Artemis acted as midwife at the birth of her own twin! You gotta love mythology.

Artemis is associated with childbirth, and while many believe this is because of the role she played at the birth of Apollo, there is more to it than that. In ancient Greece, childbearing women would pray to her before and during labor, asking her to ease the journey and save them from possible death, a somewhat common occurrence back then. She had several names and descriptors including "Locheia" (which is very similar to the word *lochia*, which is the post-birth bloody discharge that occurs when the uterus sloughs its extra lining and whose root means "pertaining to childbirth").[1] Artemis is also identified with Eileithyia, the pre-Hellenic goddess of childbirth mentioned before.[2] For the Greeks, Artemis was clearly associated with childbirth for reasons beyond her role as her mother's midwife.

Let's explore Artemis and her twin Apollo *symbolically*. As is the case with mythology, gods and goddesses can be viewed as metaphors for more than their main roles or titles suggest. Each deity is the manifestation of energies, values, and conditions present in human life. In myths and fairy tales, twins are often like two sides of the same coin—connected and complementary, but opposite. This is true of the twins Apollo and Artemis, who work as a useful metaphor for contemporary birth.

Apollo is the most favored son of Zeus and second only to him in the hearts of the Greeks. As a sun god, he is known as Phoebus Apollo, meaning "bright one." As the god of prophecy, Apollo is seen as the one who knows and understands and is therefore associated with knowledge. He is also known as the interpreter and upholder of law and order as well as the bringer of plagues and the god of healing. He is also connected to symbols of culture as the god of music and poetry.

Apollo prefers order, objectivity, and control as well as unambiguous definitions, clarity, and light that leaves little in the shadows. He dislikes chaos or passionate intensity, preferring order and structure—hence

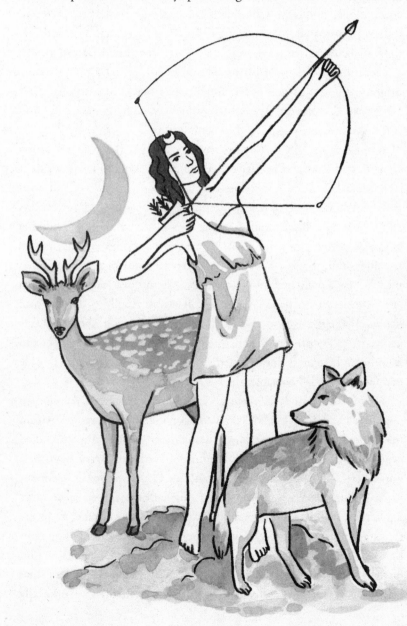

his love of laws and political structures that are meant to give society stability and harmony.

Apollo represents much of what is most revered within Western culture today, including order, control, logical thinking, intellectual knowledge, time, civilization, the ability to determine the future, youthfulness, and light. Childbirth is not exempt from these preferred values. In an Apollonian society, order, time, predictability, and civilized social behavior reign supreme. Consider the characteristics of the location where most births take place—hospitals. Hospitals are brightly lit, sterile, well-ordered, and hierarchical institutions. They are nearly temples to Apollonian values. Which makes sense, too, since Apollo is the patron god of medicine!

Artemis is the yin to Apollo's yang. Artemis is the huntress in the wilderness, friend and hunter of wild animals. Artemis favors instinct, impulse, and natural order. She can be vicious, impulsive, and swift acting. Artemis feels rather than thinks. She is the wild to Apollo's cultured and civilized order. Artemis lives in the wilderness while her twin lives within cities and towns. She is most at home with the animal creatures of the forest, while Apollo prefers the company of well-cultured men. Where Apollo is at home in the sky, Artemis lives close to the earth and is *of* the earth. If he is order, she is chaos. Apollo is the day, and Artemis the night. Where he is social and loves attention, she is viciously protective of her privacy. Where Apollo is reason, Artemis is instinct and impulse. Where he is linear, orderly, and directive, she is unpredictable and hidden. He is knowable; she is mysterious.

Society and modern medical establishments revere Apollonian qualities, but what about birth? Left alone, childbirth resides within the unpredictable and animalistic domain of Artemis. The embodied experience of birth—the animal nature of birth—is Artemisian. It is unpredictable like a storm and yet rhythmic like the waves in the ocean. Artemis values darkness, privacy, and being left undisturbed, as do birthing bodies. Birth is not lofty and tidy as Apollo prefers, but close to the earth, grounded, and messy like the wilderness that is Artemis's domain. Birth follows the strange order of nature that can look like chaos. And birth is an experience close to the deep reality of being human—that place that reminds us we can be wounded, potentially even mortally.

Apollo, as a worshiper of youth, prefers to keep the truth of mortality hidden away from the activity of everyday life.

What do these two ancient deities have to do with birth today? They beautifully exemplify the opposing forces at play in all births in today's society—regardless of whether you birth in a hospital or next to a stream in the woods. In essence, birthing takes place in an Artemisian body within an Apollonian cultural setting. The inner landscape is Artemisian while the outer, cultural landscape, is Apollonian. Understanding these two energies helps to better understand the clash and the benefits of both sides of the contemporary birthing coin.

The mythic message of birth from Artemis is about power, not control—power like that of wild Artemis. She is powerful and one with the wilderness . . . some say she *is* the wilderness. One aspect of that power includes *surrendering* to the experience itself, regardless of the path the birth takes. This letting go includes the loss of an idealized image of birth, a release of the proverbial or literal candles and flowing nightgowns. Without being aware of it, even the natural birth movement bought into the idea that there is an objective truth to right birthing. Birth entered the order-revering realm of Apollo and moved away from the subjectivity, chaos, and wild, out-of-control energy where Artemis resides.

Try This

Connecting with Artemis's Realm

To expand your ability to sit in the wild and unpredictable elements of Artemis's realm, try these suggestions:

- Consciously choose to regularly unplug from technology.

- Try connecting with your unborn baby in less technological ways like meditation, visualization, and belly touch.

- Keep a dream journal or simply pay attention to your dreams. Pregnancy dreams can be very interesting!

- Get out in nature.

The Chemistry of Labor

Hormones in pregnancy, labor, and postpartum are complex and *important*. While there are many hormones at work during this time, I'm going to simplify and focus on those that are most relevant and how they relate to our discussion of the Apollonian and Artemisian aspects of birth.

The hormonal changes in a birthing person's body while pregnant shift the brain away from issues of organization, sedating their otherwise productive brain and opening it toward a more intuitive knowing.[3] This move by nature can be shocking and deeply unsettling, exemplified by the common euphemism "pregnancy brain," meant in a derogatory manner to refer to the inability of this altered brain to function as effectively within Apollonian culture. In this way, nature reminds us that we are not only humans, but humans driven by hormones.

Neuropsychiatrist Louann Brizendine explains this movement away from linear abstraction toward an intuitive felt-sense in relation to the hormonal bath washing over the pregnant parent. "Progesterone spikes from ten to a hundred times its normal levels during the first two to four months of pregnancy, and the brain becomes marinated in the hormone, whose sedating effects are similar to those of the drug Valium."[4] The natural process of pregnancy actively sedates the pregnant parent's brain. It may not be as easy for someone pregnant to engage in the purpose-focused processes that have previously defined their life. This can be very confusing and disheartening for someone used to being a high-functioning member of a predominantly Apollonian society where productivity is highly valued.

Toward late pregnancy, stress hormones increase, making a pregnant person vigilant about their "safety, nutrition, and surroundings, and less attuned to other kinds of tasks, such as making conference calls and organizing" their schedule.[5] The animal nature of the pregnant body shifts attention from the modern foci on linear analytic thought and action toward nurturing and tending to the survival of offspring. In this way, the so-called "mommy brain" is functional in an Artemisian, nature-focused, body-centered way. It is only *dysfunctional* in how it hinders action in modern, technological, thought-centered, Apollonian society. It is this movement that pregnant people often sense intuitively in response to their observations of what is occurring in their bodies. Thanks in part to their hormones, pregnant parents begin to feel a pull inward.

Pregnancy is a preparation for birth and new parenthood, and the hormonal cocktail increases in complexity as labor begins. While progesterone was high in pregnancy, it collapses in labor, and oxytocin begins its job, contracting the uterus.

Oxytocin

Oxytocin is often referred to as the "love hormone," as it is the primary hormone responsible for coupling and falling in love and is the hormone that expands the blood vessels after orgasm, giving you a rosy afterglow. It is also the hormone responsible for contracting the uterus during labor and after birth, and it also aids in lactation. It is sometimes joked that what it took to get the baby in is what is needed to get the baby out—oxytocin plays an important role in each. Oxytocin is as responsible for the contractions and the discomfort they cause as it is for the sense of love and the experience of orgasm.

Oxytocin is released from the pituitary gland in patterned pulses.[6] Interestingly, one of the differences between oxytocin and the synthetic form of oxytocin given in hospitals to induce or augment labor, known by the brand names Pitocin and Syntocinon, is the way it's administered—intravenously or intramuscularly rather than in pulses.[7] This could be one reason the body might respond differently to naturally occurring oxytocin than it does to external supplementation—including more intense contractions. But that might not be the only reason supplemented oxytocin doesn't always increase contractions or aid in dilation of the cervix. There is another important factor in the body's use of oxytocin.

The pituitary gland releases oxytocin, but *oxytocin receptors* must be available to receive the hormone for it to effectively create contractions. These receptors in the uterine wall increase twelvefold from early pregnancy to the last weeks of pregnancy, peak at birth, and then drop significantly after birth.[8] When inductions fail to produce an effective labor, it could be due to low numbers of receptors to receive the supplemental oxytocin even when a lot has been administered.[9]

Contractions brought on by oxytocin usually create a sensation most people call pain. This pain and intensity trigger the brain to respond.

Endorphins

The body releases neurochemicals called "endorphins" in response to the multitude of experiences associated with labor. Again, I'm simplifying for ease of understanding. Chances are you've experienced the effects of endorphins when you've exercised, been stressed, or become excited. Endorphins work like an opiate such as morphine. In fact, the word *endorphin* is related etymologically to the French word *endorphine* which was coined in the 1970s using *endo*, meaning "grows within" and *morphine*.[10] Endorphins reduce the sensations of pain and discomfort while also helping the body to relax.

Endorphins increase in relation to being needed. They act as nature's response to pain. Oxytocin and endorphins are wrapped in a tightly linked dance: the more oxytocin, the more contractions; the more contractions, the more pain; the more pain, the more endorphins released in response to the pain. Sounds good, right? We feel pain and our body sends naturally occurring morphine. What could be better?

Sadly, endorphins lag behind pain, only sometimes giving relief in equal proportion to the pain. There is usually a differential between the pain and the relief offered by the pain-relieving endorphins. As pain intensifies, so does the rate of endorphins being released. But there is usually a gap between them that frequently results in feeling pain even

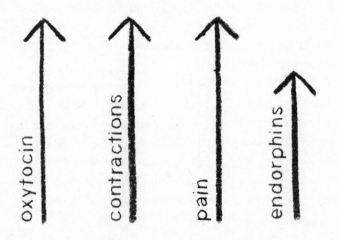

when endorphins are flowing. Some of the most intense periods of labor happen when pain spikes, but endorphins have plateaued in response to pain at a lower intensity level, making the difference stark. Many times those intense periods require parents to hold on through the plateau while the endorphins catch up.

Endorphins build over time. Later in labor the quantity of endorphins in your body is greater than it was early in labor, thus helping you cope at this higher intensity level. But that also means that if you remove the pain with an epidural and then decide to turn it down later in labor in order to have more sensation for pushing or birth, the intensity of the contractions has continued to increase, but your experience of pain has not. Therefore, your body has not needed to continue to release endorphins at the rate needed to help manage pain. When this happens, the intensity felt when the pain meds are turned down can be completely overwhelming and feel far *worse* than when the epidural was administered.

The role of endorphins in response to pain is somewhat familiar, especially to athletes. These hormones are predominantly responsible for creating the euphoric feeling that often follows a hard workout, the so-called "runner's high." Endorphins create a similar "high" in labor producing the otherworldly, trance-like state often experienced by those deep in labor. In this way, endorphins help you soften around the intensity of labor, cope with the physical and emotional challenges, and reduce stress and fear. This response loop is a delicate one: more oxytocin invites more endorphins (to a point), and more endorphins signals the brain to release more.

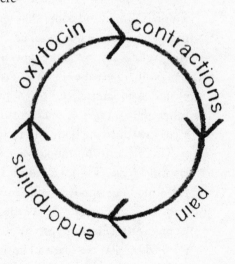

Remember the metaphor of the train with regard to labor in the previous chapter? In many ways, oxytocin is the fuel for the train. Without enough of it, the train is unlikely to go anywhere. The whole cycle—oxytocin, contractions, pain, endorphins, and back to oxytocin—has to spin for the train to get going. Disrupt any of the elements—including pain—too early in the process, and the train may slow down or go off the tracks. This wheel is a cycle where each element influences the flow of the other. It is a biofeedback loop. Remove something as seemingly insignificant to the *function* of the cycle like pain, and the brain may not continue to get the signal to release oxytocin. This is one of the reasons that epidurals given early in labor (before six centimeters) often slow down labor, and Pitocin is used to get labor moving again. It can take a long time for the body to get into the groove of labor. Getting the labor train really moving down the tracks before removing anything from the cycle, including pain, can help labor function effectively.

Inner Landscape of Birth

Together, oxytocin and endorphins create a unique inner landscape within the mind and body. They send the laboring parent inward where they often become less social or Apollonian. Oxytocin, with its associated feelings of love and connection and the accompanying physical sensations, draws the laboring person toward the Artemisian attributes of intuition, nature, and body. The endorphin bath adds to this, diffusing the experience, often creating a hazy perception that turns all focus inward to the body and the totality of the sensory experience.

This delicate hormonal dance occurs totally unnoticed by the laboring person's rational mind. In this hormonal haze there is little place for more modern constructs such as linear time, intellectual reason, or even language. As this shift in consciousness occurs, the labor can feel like an entirely different land, otherworldly or "out there." I think it is a place all its own, and I love the term "Laborland" used by Pam England and others to identify this unique inner landscape.[11] This emotional, physical, spiritual place in birth is entirely another realm.

THE BIRTHING BRAIN

While the brain is a highly complex organ that defies simplification, I am going to do exactly that—simplify it. This is not a book about neuroscience; what we really need to know concerns what happens in the brain during birth and why it matters. It is generally agreed upon by neuroscientists that the brain has an older more primitive brain structure responsible for basic survival functions and a newer brain structure responsible for more cognitive functions.

The "old brain" includes, among other things, the hypothalamus. Its key function is to help the body maintain homeostasis, playing a key role in regulating hunger, thirst, body temperature, sleep cycles, sex drive, and . . . childbirth. Critical for our purposes is to know that oxytocin is produced in the hypothalamus and released by the pituitary gland—both part of the older brain.

Let's circle back to Artemis. Remember that Artemis's energies are those of the wild rather than of culture. She is all about the instinctual nature, the autonomic systems, the act-before-you-think way of living. As the goddess of the wilderness, Artemis respects cycles like those of the seasons, the moon, day and night, and sleep and waking. She also respects the impulses of animals such as the need to drink and eat as well as the drive to reproduce. Do you see the connection I'm making here? Artemis represents the aspects of the brain regulated by the older part, which could be called the "Artemisian brain."

Now let's look at the neocortex, or new brain. This part of the brain is responsible for what we think of as higher functions such as conscious thought, reasoning, sense perception, and language. Yep, that's the Apollonian brain! Apollo is the god who is all about the things that differentiate cultured society from the wilderness, including rational thought, critical thinking, and language. Apollo's realm begins at the edge of civilization in terms of both society and the brain. Apollo respects order, reason, and knowledge, and as the god of poetry—language.

Artemis represents the hormonal aspects of birth governed by the hormones released from the old brain, and Apollo represents the activity of the new brain. Both the old brain and the new brain play important, and sometimes oppositional, roles in human birth. Here's where it gets really interesting. You need to go into the old brain, the instinctual brain, your Artemisian brain, to trigger and maintain the flow of oxytocin. In order to do this, you have to connect with all those parts that exist within Artemis's wilderness.

Apollo's realm and all its characteristics such as bright light, social engagement, language, and rational thought activate the neocortex, which can negatively affect the activity in the old brain. We humans frequently use our thinking mind to influence our instinctual mind. Take sex for example. Most of us have at some point talked ourselves into or out of sexual arousal. Want to get in the mood? Watching a romantic movie or talking about sexual fantasies often engage the thinking mind in an effort to excite sexual arousal. Thoughts are also often used to suppress unwanted arousal, especially for men who don't want their excitement to be visually obvious. People sometimes try to think their way out of arousal by engaging thoughts about things like sports, their parents, or other unsexy things. Similarly, we may not be hungry, but if we talk about food, see food, or even think about that great meal we had recently, the body may start to actually feel the need to eat. The instinctual brain can, and often is, influenced by conscious thoughts.

What does this mean in labor? Our modern mode of birth is highly dominated by symbols that activate the conscious mind. Hospitals are brightly lit, populated by strangers, packed with hard angles and lines rather than softer edges like those found in nature, filled with the sounds of machines and voices rather than of water or wind, and perhaps most challenging, organized around clock time rather than the cycles of nature. Is it any wonder that so many labors need to be augmented by synthetic oxytocin to keep things moving? The neocortex is overly stimulated in such an environment, and the instinctual brain as a result may go quiet.

Creating an Environment for Labor

Regardless of where you give birth, keep Artemis and the characteristics of her environment in mind as you create a space conducive to birthing.

Darkness

Turn off the lights. Most hospital rooms have *a lot* of lighting options. There are usually main lights, under-cabinet lighting, wall sconces, a spot light for stitching and other procedures that require close visual inspection, bathroom lights, and even dim lighting that comes from the machines in the room. Which lights are really needed, and which ones can you turn off to help bring more of a nighttime energy into the room? You can also bring battery-operated candles or twinkly lights to create a warmer glow to the atmosphere. Some parents wear dark sunglasses to carry the dimmed lighting with them wherever they go. One client told me that after her birth, she looked at some photos of her labor, and there she was . . . completely naked except for her shades!

Privacy

Artemis does not like to be observed. One myth tells of how she discovered that she was being watched by a hunter while she bathed. This invasion of her privacy made her so angry that she turned the voyeur into a stag and had him hunted to death by his own hounds. The myths of what happens to mortals who observe Artemis are a bit horrifying but do communicate the point of how much she does not like to be observed! This desire for privacy is true of the laboring brain as well.

What can you do to create a more private place for your labor?

Close the door to your room. Strange as it may seem, it is common to see doors open on labor floors in hospitals. A simple sign that communicates a lot to your mind and to those around you is a closed door. Hospital staff will still check on you, and, if monitors are being used, they can see the data they gather in another area. Some parents even put a sign on the door with their request for privacy and their wish that anyone coming in knock first.

Parents craving privacy may find the bathroom to be their favorite nesting place. Restrooms are special places for a number of reasons. First, we are used to being alone in a bathroom (unless you have a toddler, then you're never used to using the bathroom by yourself). Second, in bathrooms we're used to doing things we wouldn't normally do in public—we see these rooms as places of privacy. Third, bathrooms are frequently windowless so they're easier to get dark than a large labor room with big windows. And finally, bathrooms are generally small, making it more difficult for lots of people to gather in one—although I've seen a bathroom fill with people when a birth is imminent. Here's a pro tip for you: bring battery-operated lighting of some sort as the florescent lights in the bathroom are often the only option, and they're very bright!

Many hospitals in my area boast about their beautiful windows during tours of the labor ward. As beautiful as the view might be, one of the first things most parents do when they arrive in their labor room is to close the curtains!

Another option for at least a *sense* of privacy is to create a portable space that feels semiprivate. Have you ever been to a coffee shop and looked around the crowd? You know right away who is not interested in talking to anyone because they have on sunglasses and headphones. This body language says to everyone, "I'm not open for conversation." You can create this same small private space for yourself during labor. Doing so can be very helpful, especially during the transition from home to hospital or birth center. Fewer people will try to engage with you if you're wearing the universal signs of "I don't want to talk!"

Warmth

If you've ever seen a cat or a dog give birth, they tend to find the most out of the way, private, dark, warm place possible . . . sometimes in the basket with clean clothes that have just come out of the drier. People in labor also crave privacy, darkness, and warmth. Most people in labor need to be warm but then can get too hot during contractions. It is common to see a person in labor curled up or walking around in a warm blanket, robe, or sweater, only to throw it off when a contraction starts. Then, after the contraction has passed, they feel cold and need warmth again during the rest period. One of my favorite amenities at a hospital or birth center is the seemingly endless supply of warmed blankets that no one in your family has to launder!

Smells

Our sense of smell is a powerful one that connects deeply to our memory circuits in the brain. Most medical establishments smell, well, medical.

They may smell like cleaning supplies, disinfectants, alcohol, and other clinical scents. Some people are bothered by these smells and want to have a more pleasant scent instead. Some parents like to bring scented lotion, massage oil, or essential oils to use to help mask the smell with something more pleasing. Be careful. Many people in labor are *very* sensitive to smells, and a pleasant scent can become irritating if too much is used. Three favorite fragrances in labor are lavender, peppermint, and chamomile.

Cyclical Time

Rather than paying attention to clock time, allow the cycle of the day to wax and wane. Cover up clocks or turn your attention away from them and onto the flow of the experience. Few people who labor without pain medication can tell their labor story according to a timeline. Instead, labor is remembered as a series of events that link together in some way that is reminiscent to the memory of a dream we've had. There is a tendency for parents to time contractions as soon as they start and to do so with a visible stopwatch, clock, or phone. Reduce the use of clocks as much as possible. Only bring out something to time contractions if what you *see* makes you want confirmation of the sort that a clock can give. As much as possible, adjust to the idea that time in labor moves differently—more organically and less predictably. Time in labor is Artemisian; it's connected to the cycles of nature rather than a clock.

Clock time is Apollonian and often used in labor in an attempt to turn something that is unpredictable and seemingly irrational into something well-ordered and reliable. Birth according to clock time inspires doing *something* rather than waiting for birth to do what it needs to do. Waiting is counter to action, which holds a higher value in Western culture than observation. It is believed that to do something is better than doing nothing. Additionally, clock time adds to the myth of control by creating units that are easily measured between events, thus mimicking order and predictability, while also giving progress the *appearance* of linearity and appeasing the Apollonian cultural value.

While graphs and clocks continue to define birth progress from a linear, rational, external perspective, birthing parents continue to experience birth in an internal, hazy way that is not able to be located within clock time. The emotional experience of birth exists in a difficult-to-define period rarely experienced through clock time. When new parents share their experience of labor with others shortly after their birth, they often start the story with the time their labor began. From there, rarely do they remember the movement of their labor with time stamps until the time the baby is born. It is only with the help or influence of those there with them that birthing people place their birth experience within an ordered time-based narrative. Birthing parents expecting to follow the progression of their labor through attachment to clock time may keep themselves from dropping into the mammalian, body-centered Artemisian process that aids in the functional hormonal progression.

Technology

As much as possible, reduce the visible or obtrusive use of technology in labor. This includes or is perhaps *mostly* about cell phones. Turn all phones off or put them in silent mode. Keep them tucked away and out of sight. If using them for photos, do so in a subtle and noninvasive way. TVs and computers too can be activating for the neocortex. While settling into a good movie during early labor can be a great way to relax and slow down, once labor progresses, it's best to reduce the presence of technological devices.

In hospital labor rooms, technological devices are set up throughout the space. As much as you are able, focus your attention on other things that help you soften and settle into your body. Close your eyes, or if they're open, focus on things like photos of loved ones or beloved pets, the flickering of a candle (battery-operated of course), or even better, the eyes of your beloved. Partners, rather than using the monitor to tell when your beloved is having a contraction, watch them to see when a contraction starts to roll in by the way they move their body, change their facial expression, or make sounds. These signs are often subtler and require being in tune with your partner in a way that the contraction monitor does not. That's the point! Staying deeply connected will help your beloved as they go through contractions.

Intimacy

Remember that the instinctual brain controls functions beyond birth and includes sexual arousal. Maintain or create an environment that supports your intimate connection with your beloved. Use eye gazing, kissing, loving words, massage, tender and sensual touch, and other physical signs of affection that help create and maintain a sense of intimacy between you. Follow the laboring person's desires regarding what forms of sensual connection work for them. Some people don't like to be touched at all in labor while others wish to be enveloped in their lover's arms.

Movement

An environment that encourages movement is beneficial. Being able to freely move around, shift and change positions, and walk can help labor. Have you ever used one of those plastic sifters at the beach? You load it up with sand and if you hold it still, very little falls out. You have to shake it to help the sand find its way through the holes. This is like your baby finding its way through your pelvis. The pelvis is a relatively tight passage, and your baby's head is a relatively large mass to get through that tight space. When attempting to fit something through a tight space, lubricants often help. Think of motion as a lubricant to help baby move down and through your pelvis. An easy way to remember this is "motion is lotion." Silly perhaps, but memorable!

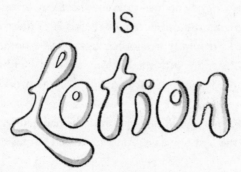

MOTION IS Lotion

Emotion

The other lubricant for labor is the open flow of emotions. Make sure your environment supports the free release of your emotions. Holding back tears, upset, or other strong emotions is, in essence, closing. In labor, remember, we want to focus on opening. Open, open, open. That includes opening to your emotions as they come. Tears are sometimes said to be a lubricant for labor. Let them flow rather than holding them back. Welcome them. Like motion, emotion is lotion as well.

There are two other elements that we have to address in our exploration of how the brain works in labor: stress and fear.

Stress

Why is the environment for labor so important? We have to return to our discussion of brain chemistry. Remember that for labor to progress smoothly, oxytocin has to flow. According to neuroeconomist, Paul Zak, "High stress blocks oxytocin release," which makes sense when you consider that oxytocin "drives empathic concern (compassion)—which might get in the way of fighting for your life."[12] This means that as stress and/or fear go up, the release of oxytocin goes down. If oxytocin drops during labor, contractions can slow or stop, and labor will either slow or stall as a result. In most cases when this happens, rather than address the cause of stress, many medical providers supplement labor by adding external oxytocin in the form of Pitocin.

A birthing parent who feels inhibited in labor may not feel safe to labor down and birth their baby. Vigilant awareness supplied by the stress hormones drops only when a laboring person feels a sense of safety. The trouble is in determining what supports the concept of safety, as it is not clearly defined or even objectively definable. For one person, it might be the most state-of-the-art hospital with the most highly regarded doctors. For another, it might be home alone with no one else to interfere with the birthing process. Neither is right or wrong; they just depend on the individual. Regardless, it's good to know how this system works.

Amanda's labor is a good case in point. She had a long, slow start to her labor. For the first few days, Amanda stayed home, ate, slept, and moved around, but real active labor was rather illusive. Her intended birth location was a small community hospital about an hour away without traffic (a rare occurrence in this part of Los Angeles) and much farther away with more difficult road conditions. On day three of her slow, start-stop labor, Amanda declared it was time to go to the hospital. As a birth attendant, it was pretty clear to me that her labor was not at the point where being at the hospital was necessary, at least not yet. But when a laboring mama says, "Let's go," you go! Her birth team loaded into various cars and headed over the hill. It did take over an hour to get there, and Amanda was checked at the clinic confirming what I suspected: there wasn't much cervical dilation. She was given the choice to head back home or check into the hospital. With the prospect of another hour or more drive home and a return trip at some later time, Amanda chose to check into the hospital. Curiously, it wasn't long after she checked in that things started to progress. It was as if her labor was waiting for her to settle into the hospital before it kicked into higher gear! Could it be that Amanda's stress hormones were keeping vigilant guard until she felt safe to let down and settle into more active labor?

Amanda's story is not unique. I have witnessed labors that had stalled at home reinvigorate upon crossing the threshold of the hospital. No one location provides a *universal* sense of safety.

The more common example of when this protective function goes into effect is visible when labors in high gear at home slow or stop when parents arrive at the hospital. This could be the brain's way of protecting the laboring person from the perceived threat it has registered due to the unfamiliar surroundings. Believe it or not, this is the body's built-in protection system doing what it's meant to do!

In prehistoric times, this innate system protected our ancestors and their offspring from predators. If a prehistoric woman in labor sensed a threat, two key events would happen to help keep her safe: one, her labor would slow so that her baby would not be born in the presence of a threat, and two, the stress hormones pumping through her system would bring clarity to her mind quickly so that she could use the best weapon she had against a predator—her big brain and its ability to think of a way out.

As is often the case with natural functions, it does not always work in as simplified a way as I have been describing. There is more to stress hormones and labor. Sometimes a rush of a stress hormone, such as adrenaline, has the opposite effect on labor and can actually increase the pace of the process. Thinking back to the prehistoric mother, a high release of stress hormones near the end of birth might aid in the speedy expulsion of her baby, which in turn could help protect the mother and child from a threat like a saber-toothed tiger. When a baby is near to birth, the pelvic floor bulges between the legs. Imagine for a moment, having to walk, let alone *run* with a baby's head bulging between your thighs! In situations where the labor is already too far along to stop, it might be better for the parent to birth the child quickly than to stop the process.

Another place where variations are normal is in the birthing parent's reaction immediately following birth. While some parents have a rush of euphoria and excitedly reach for their baby, this doesn't always happen. Regardless of what the images shared on social media seem to communicate, some parents who have just gone through the intensity of labor and birth are not really on the planet right after. It could be said that these parents are so deeply *in* their bodies that they need a moment or two to return to the world around them before they can even show interest in their baby. This moment of deep internal relief of "Oh my God, I survived," is a normal response that says nothing about the love the parent has for their new baby. Let this post-birth pause happen without judgment or haste. At some point, the birthing parent will return and be ready to bond.

A spike in stress hormones just before the urge to push can also cause birthing parents to experience and express fear. For many experienced birth attendants, this statement of doubt is viewed as a telltale sign that the time of birth is approaching. Remember that the body releases stress hormones in response to doubt or fear, and this hormonal shift gives the laboring parent greater clarity, focus, and strength, all of which are valuable for the effort required to birth a baby. This shift out of the laboring fog of Laborland can also help ready the new parent to meet and tend to the newborn baby.

If fear and doubt can trigger a hormonal reaction in the body that can either inhibit the progress of labor or speed it up, how is it possible to know which response the body will have to stressful external stimuli? Like so many things in nature, there is no way to know conclusively. The biology of birth is veiled in a lot of mystery, making it difficult to understand, predict, or control.

Fear

All of this discussion of stress hormones can leave parents wondering how they can reduce fear and its accompanying hormones so as to not hinder birth. My teacher, Pam, says, "Worry is the work of pregnancy."[13] I believe this to be true. There are few events that elicit worry and anxiety like becoming pregnant and facing the unfamiliar landscapes of labor, birth, and impending parenthood. Fear and anxiety are normal parts of pregnancy.

> Birth doesn't ask you to be fearless. It asks you to be brave.

I do not believe that the goal of birth is to be fearless. Instead, I believe birth requires courage. There's a huge difference between the two. Being fearless implies a *lack* of fear, whereas being courageous means that even if fear comes, we can *still* move forward in the face of it.

The wilderness of birth can be an anxiety-producing place. To remove all fear is to impose Apollonian rules on Artemis's realm. The wilderness resists such conformity. Still, there are things we can do to address our concerns so that we reduce the possibility that stress-producing events occur. We will explore fear further later on. Up next is how to face that Big Bad Wolf—pain.

The Four-Letter Word

No exploration about childbirth would be complete without a discussion of pain. The avoidance of pain is not exclusive to childbirth; rather, it is woven into the very fabric of being human. We are conditioned to believe that any inkling of pain is an indication that something is wrong and needs to be fixed. In most instances, this is true. If we stub a toe or break a bone, the pain we feel gives us information about what is happening to our body and inspires us to do something about it. When we feel the pain of a blister forming in our hiking boot, that pain lets us know we need to stop and protect the hotspot from further irritation. This mental programing helps protect our bodies from harm. We feel pain, and we act to do something about it.

On the other side, we've heard the more modern adage, "no pain, no gain" tossed around on sports fields and in athletic gyms. This idea reinforces the belief that without a bit of discomfort, we won't develop new skills and stronger muscles.

Strangely, neither of these beliefs, conditioned or learned, completely apply to the pain, discomfort, hard work, and intensity that accompanies the birth of a baby. The physical pain is caused by the tightening of uterine muscles and the stretching of the cervix as it pulls back and opens enough for a baby to pass through. The effort, work, and stretch these muscles go through is what causes much of the pain associated with labor contractions. Unlike the pain experienced with a broken bone, this pain is not meant to inform the brain that something is wrong. Instead, it is pain with a purpose.

Perhaps labor pain is closer to that experienced in a tough athletic workout where pain derives from muscles working hard and stretching in new ways. However, the energy of pushing through the pain that we often rely on to get through a difficult physical workout is not what usually best supports labor.

You may also have heard that labor does not *have* to be painful. There is a movement in the birth world about rebranding labor pain as intensity or discomfort and renaming contractions rushes, surges, or waves. I've even seen contractions renamed "baby hugs."[1] I understand the desire behind this effort at rebranding—to change the experience by changing our understanding of it in the first place. But there is an undesirable side effect of doing this: we have stopped preparing for the truth of just how hard giving birth can be. I have heard of and spoken with many parents who head into birth grasping hold of the idea that labor will be intense or challenging, but not painful. When labor is a reality rather than an imaginary future event, these parents are often bowled over by the physical discomfort that can only be called pain.

It is not enough to redefine pain. We must expand our ideas about what the many different experiences might be in labor *and* build our capacity to handle whatever labor or postpartum gives us to deal with. It is my desire to help you become stronger in the face of pain and intensity. We have been taught that any hint of pain, even in conversation, is to be eliminated as if it were the most ultimate of evils. Pain is culturally vilified. If we hold the idea that saying the word *pain* will cause it to be true, we give immense power to pain. It becomes the Voldemort of childbirth.[2]

Remember, in the world of the Harry Potter novels and movies most witches and wizards won't even say the Dark Lord's name. In refusing to do so, Voldemort is imbued with more awe and fear than he truly deserves. Dumbledore understood this and said to Harry: "Call him Voldemort, Harry. Always use the proper name for things.

Fear of a name increases fear of the thing itself."[3] So, too, with pain in labor. We need to be Harry here and call pain by its name, thus removing its mysterious otherworldly power to elicit fear. So what if labor is painful? You are strong.

Additionally, no one definition or singular description can harness all that the experience of pain is. Pain is utterly subjective and personal, which makes defining it challenging. The idea of pain having a universal quality, even in the general experience of childbirth, is impossible or at least foolish. Each individual person experiences painful sensations in different ways, including variations with respect to intensity, pressure, texture, and duration.

The sensations of labor are too big, varied, and multidimensional to capture in a single word. Labor sensations are often painful *and* intense, as well as potentially fatiguing, hard, challenging, gripping, tightening, crampy, opening, fluid, strong, and so much more.

In addition, labor is a larger and more all-encompassing experience that cannot be reduced to the sensations of the body alone. Labor is far more than any single four-letter word can convey. Let's not cloak it in euphemisms. Labor can be physically painful, and emotionally intense, and challenging on relationships, and highly spiritual, and mentally demanding, and joyful beyond comprehension, and a hold-on-by-your-fingernails roller-coaster ride, and an ecstatic, heart-bursting, love-filled experience. It can be all of those and more! And, it can be all of those *at the same time!*

THE VILIFICATION OF PAIN

Cultural messages about conquering are common around pain. Pain, we have learned, is a villain that needs to be defeated. In a culture that is ever focused on advancement, domination, and control, pain is seen as yet another obstacle to surmount. Don't get me wrong; I'm human and I don't like pain and suffering any more than the next person. I try hard to avoid unnecessary suffering. And yet, as a birth professional for over twenty years, I've seen that our cultural abhorrence of pain often causes more suffering than if we were prepared for and open to the painful aspects of birth.

Pain reminds us of our mortality, our existence in bodily matter. It reminds us not only that we are humans, but that as humans we are also animals. It thrusts us into sharp awareness that Apollo's culture is not the only side of the coin. Pain, physical or otherwise, often causes us to revert to a nonverbal state. To be reduced to grunts and moans is to face our animal selves head on. It plunges us deep into the wilderness of Artemis's realm. Pain in labor compels us to communicate without civilized words, to communicate as animals do—lowering us from our hierarchically superior position of civilized human to that of "lowly" animals. This reversal of status is seen as undesirable, uncultured, and, to most modern Western people, unnecessary.

Some argue that our ability to remove pain is part of what makes us civilized. Except, pain is part of life. What then is lost when pain is devalued, removed, or suppressed? Pain gives us the valley side of the emotional experience that, by its existence, helps to shape our emotional peaks and in so doing, our humanity. It is in contrast to pain, at least in part, that we are able to experience sensations of joy and love.

To think of pain as a puzzle to solve engages the civilized self, the part of us that believes there are rational fixes to any problem—Apollo's realm. From that perspective, pain needs to be fixed and understood, the puzzle needs to be completed. But when pain is explored instead through the lens of mystery, then it falls more comfortably into the realm of the unknowable, inexplicable, and wild—the land of Artemis. As such, pain may actually be functional during situations that demand an altered state of consciousness, like rites of passage. To view pain as functional unsettles our cultural understanding of it and challenges the meaning we give it.

It is so deeply imbedded in our unconscious to do something about pain and to resist becoming an animal in the face of it, that almost all births in the United States today are supported by pharmaceutical pain-relieving measures—most often epidurals. Medical science is miraculous, and its ability to prevent unnecessary suffering is an incredible gift to humankind. However, in birth, interventions that reduce or eliminate intense pain can sometimes suppress the body's ability to go through the physical changes necessary to birth. And since pain and loss are integral parts of many rites of passage, might suppressing all pain actually deprive or delay the birthing parent's successful psychological transformation from individual to parent?

The medical model is not alone in its response to cultural influences and judgments around pain. The natural birth model also has judgments about pain.

Many birth professionals agree that the natural birth movement began with Dr. Grantly Dick-Read. His philosophy was grounded in the idea that pain was a negative and destructive force in labor that should be conquered by removing fear, since according to Dick-Read, fear creates pain.[4] There are movements that have taken this even farther, where the goal of a pain-free birth is no longer enough. Now we must aim for an orgasmic birth. I do believe that orgasmic births happen. What I don't believe is that believing in them means you will get one.

Threaded throughout the natural birth movement are similar associations to, and even denial of, pain. One common belief goes something like this: "If you believe there will be no pain strongly enough and truly enough, you will not experience it." This relationship to and vilification of pain puts the responsibility squarely in the birthing parent's hands. It is as if to say, if you do it "right," you will be free from pain. You just need to trust *enough*. One of the unintended side effects of having this much responsibility is the guilt that can come from failing to achieve the wished-for experience of a pain-free birth. Here, "mother guilt" starts early.

I see the denial of pain repeatedly in the parents who come to my classes. This thread runs deeply through the natural birth community and is reinforced by the slogans, "Birth is beautiful" and "Your body was made to do this." Both birth mantras put pain in the back seat and create instead an image of beauty and ease. It is from this denial of pain and its replacement with beauty that we get the labors that are all candles and flowing white nightgowns, and where pain and even hard work are uninvited guests. Sadly, when they do show up, they are so unexpected they can ruin the whole party. Labor requires far more from a person than positive affirmations. Unfortunately, the denial of pain often leaves parents unprepared for the whole spectrum of what labor can demand—from ecstasy to agony.

CULTIVATING COURAGE AND DEVELOPING NEW SKILLS

One of the most important things you can do to cultivate readiness for childbirth and parenthood is to expand your capacity to sit with discomfort and learn to let it flow *through* you. Some call this coping, and sometimes that's exactly what it is. But coping also elicits images and energies of holding on, gripping, clenching, and white-knuckling. Additionally, coping communicates doing and acting rather than *allowing*, which is often what's really needed in labor. While there are moments in labor (and certainly in parenthood) where coping is perhaps the best we can hope for, let's start with *being* rather than *doing*.

Most pain-coping exercises are about doing—what you can *do* to cope and get through the contraction. This makes sense, since as modern people we are most familiar and comfortable when there is something specific that can be done in the face of challenge. But to flow through labor and parenthood well, you need something beyond effort. What you need is openness to what *is* without clenching or straining. Remember, birth is about opening, not closing.

One of my first yoga teachers, Chuck, had sayings he would pepper throughout class. I both loved them and rolled my eyes at them in alternate moments. Still, many have stuck with me decades later. There's one that relates directly to what I'm sharing here. Chuck would say: "Soften all that is not needed. No unnecessary effort. Add nothing extra."

Letting go is often far more effective in labor than effort. Effort is the extra we don't want to add. Unlike the gym or sports field mentioned before, the pain of labor often requires a *flowing with* rather than an aggressive "no pain, no gain" or tough-it-out mentality. Instead, the "hard work" is often in surrendering and softening around the pain. However, while this sounds lovely, don't underestimate the challenge of doing so! This sort of intensity and pain with this type of helpful response is a new experience. Practicing now will help, as you'll need this skill not only for labor but for parenthood as well.

Putting It into Daily Practice

You can't expect to know how to soften around pain and intensity rather than resist it if you've rarely done so in your regular life. When confronted with the reality of labor, our bodies respond habitually. Here are some practices to help you build new habits.

Flow

Clenching around discomfort or pain in labor can counteract the energies going into opening the body. Clenching is counterproductive in labor. Practice being in a flow mode rather than in a closed clench.

> "It's easy enough to stand on the outside and say, 'You just have to let go and let the baby out.' But to let the baby out, you have to be willing to go to pieces." MAGGIE NELSON[5]

Try This

Moving to Music

Put on some music you love, something that makes you want to move, if not outright boogie! Let the music wash over you. Hear it, but don't listen to it actively, simply let it roll through and across your body and nervous system. As you feel drawn to, let yourself sway, move, and respond to the music without ideas of what that movement *should* be or look like. This is not a dance class. There is no right way to move. Practice letting go of the ideas that follow us into adulthood about our bodies and how they are supposed to move through space. If you feel yourself begin to take on rote or mechanized motions, pause and return to the music.

Life in modern society has likely created a clench inside of you like the tightly wound cord of an old wired telephone that you are not even fully aware of and that needs to unwind. Let yourself go, as if the movement is the beginning few spins of the headset as it dangles from the cord and begins to release and unwind. Let the movement find its own momentum. Pay attention to the tight places in your body. Soften these and the area around them as much as you are able but *without ambition*. You are practicing unwinding and opening, so it doesn't help to judge or make demands on your body to respond. There are few things that make us want to tighten more than someone (or ourselves) yelling, "Soften!" Practice opening even to the possibility that you will not be able to soften or release some areas. Simply noticing is a great place to begin.

Do one song or piece of music a day as a daily practice of unwinding and practicing being in the flow with your body.

Bedtime

As you lie in bed before you fall asleep, practice softening your muscles and letting go into the support of your bed.

 ## Try This

Relaxing Tense Muscles

Clench and then release various muscles of your body, starting from your neck and shoulders and working your way down toward your feet. If you find it difficult to identify softening or releasing, this is the one to practice. If you're already pretty familiar with what it takes to let go of existing tightness, then simply scan your body for tension and release it. Another option is to locate where you are *already* relaxed and free from clenching and then imagine spreading the relaxation throughout your body. Try supporting your partner to do this too. You can even practice guiding each other through this practice of letting go before you head to sleep or at other times in the day when you want to release or recharge.

Practicing with a Negative Stimulus

You need to prepare your mind and body for challenging circumstances, not just the easy ones. Labor and parenthood require more from us than the ability to relax while lying comfortably. To this end, I encourage parents to use a negative stimulus, such as holding ice, doing "keep-ups" (putting your arms out to your sides forming a *T* shape and spinning them in small circles), holding a squat, or doing all of the above at the same time. I want you to work with a negative stimulus not because any part of me believes that holding ice or circling your arms mimics childbirth! The truth is, there is no ethical way I could truly give you a sense of what labor might feel like! The negative stimulus gives your mind something to work with, something you wish weren't happening; that's its value.

 Try This

Practicing Ice "Contractions"

Ice practice is an exercise for your mind and is not about building tolerance to cold. If you were to only practice in a state of comfort, how would you know what helps you when something irritating, painful, or challenging occurs? Working with a negative stimulus makes translating your skills to labor an easier leap. And practicing together with your partner, or other support person, while holding ice gives both of you a better sense of what type of support might help best when things get tough. By practicing "contractions" this way, I want you to increase your mental capacity to flow *even with* those sensations you don't like and that you want to remove.

To get started, you'll need ice cubes, a timer, and a towel (I love cloth diapers as they are ridiculously absorbent and remind you of why you're doing this to begin with!). Both parents hold the ice and practice. Sometimes partners say, "I'm not going to be the one in pain. Why do I have to hold the ice?" While partners won't be feeling the sensations of contractions, there might be times in labor or new parenthood when they too have a negative sensation that they wish were different. The ice represents that as well. Once you have everything set up, you're ready to begin.

Time a sixty-second "contraction." During that minute don't *do* anything that you already know helps you when you're in discomfort. Just hold the ice in your hand, making sure to connect the surface of the ice to the skin of your hand. You are not resting the ice on the palm. Rather you're holding it inside a lightly closed fist so that the ice makes full contact. Do not put the ice down before the minute is up.

When the minute is over, put down the ice. How did you navigate the sensations? What did you do that helped you keep going even in moments when you didn't want to? *Notice what worked.*

Remember that I told you not to do anything? Is that really possible? No! The reality is that we gather abilities throughout our lives, arriving at this point with proven skills and tricks that help us, even when we're told not to use them. When you picked up this book you were likely looking for some tools to help you in labor and birth. I'm here to remind you that you *already have some*! Throughout your life you have developed skills, tools, and methods of support that help you in moments of stress or pain. Just because you're about to have a baby doesn't mean all those hard-earned abilities fly out the door. Those skills are with you, and you will likely use them many more times throughout your life as well as in labor and parenthood.

After returning from a trip to India in my early twenties that included practicing yoga for the first time, few things were clear in my life except that I needed to practice yoga daily. Upending my already ungrounded life, I relocated to Santa Monica so that I could work at YogaWorks and begin daily practice under the guidance of my teacher, Chuck, who I had met and connected with while in India. For years my morning routine involved a predawn drive, a very hot and sweaty nearly two-hour class, and a sponge shower in the sink at YogaWorks before beginning work for the day as general manager. Those mornings were my physical and spiritual practice, and all sorts of emotions came up. I would cry, moan, feel elated, break and be fixed, suffer and find equanimity, and through it all I just kept doing my practice and staying with my breath.

Here's the thing: it was what I learned during my mornings of yoga that carried me through my labor. I had taken childbirth classes and read lots of books, but where I went for support when I needed it was right back to what was *already familiar* to me from my life and was heavily tested in the alchemical vessel of daily practice.

Lessons don't have to come through physical activities. We learn every time we face challenging situations and keep going, be it difficult work situations, finals in school, grief and loss, or any number of other possibilities.

So, here's the big ah-ha: *you already know a lot*! You've made it this far in life. Use what you know, as it will serve you best when needed.

And you have time to add new skills, tools, and practices to your repertoire before birth. But if you want them to really support you, you need to practice them regularly so that your mind and body fall into flow without having to activate your thinking mind to do so. Practices need to become habits. It can be helpful to develop new habits or strengthen supportive older ones.

Breath

Start with the breath. If you are alive, then you are breathing, and the breath is a constant that can carry you through difficult moments. Focusing on the breath can be a great reminder to flow and let go since holding and clenching the breath is incompatible with survival. When we get tense, agitated, or stub our toe, how often does someone well-meaning tell us to breathe? You likely already do some version of this practice in your life. The breath is a go-to anchor for presence.

Try This

Breathing to Let Go

Now try another minute-long ice contraction, this time while placing your attention on your breath. Notice it. Bring your attention to your breath and follow it with your mind's eye. Pay special attention to your exhale. We are more conditioned to soften and release on the exhale. The outward breath is the breath of letting go, and letting go is key in labor. While some teachers have you change or alter your breath, I prefer to simply use the breath as a focal point without needing it to change or even deepen. As pregnancies advance, the ability to take a full . . . luxurious . . . extended . . . prolonged . . . deep breath vanishes with the ever-disappearing space in your torso, so don't torture yourself with the need to fill your lungs to bursting with each inhale. Pay attention to your breath as it is.

Set the timer for sixty seconds and hold the ice. Go!

What was helpful this time? What did you notice that was better? What made a difference? How did you do it? Try another one or two. Make changes and see what helps.

Water

Many laboring people speak profoundly about the power of water to soothe, distract, or help them ride the waves of contractions. What better place to practice flowing with sensation than in water!

🦋 Try This

Showering During Ice "Contractions"

Turn on the shower to a pleasing temperature. Have ice ready nearby. Get in the shower and hold the ice for a minute in both hands this time. Keep your hands out of the warm water as you don't want the water to melt the ice. Instead, let the water run over your body, hit your back, and move across your skin. Be with the water. Let the water and your breath become a rhythmic dance that carries you to the end of the minute. When the timer goes off, set down the ice. Rest for one minute before doing another minute-long ice contraction. Do this cycle of contraction-rest-contraction twice, then let what's left of your ice melt down the drain.

What did you notice that was helpful? What did you do or not do that made the ice contractions a little bit easier? Did you move or not move? What helped? Now, imagine being in the shower while you are in labor. What about this exercise might be helpful to you? Is there anything else you would add—music, movement, scents, touch, supportive words, or something else that might make this even better for you? Take mental notes or write it down in a journal or notebook you can take with you to birth (or write it in the margins here . . . I write in my books all the time).

Purposeful Distractions and Tools for Focus

Only give labor as much attention as it demands from you. If you focus too intensely on labor before that level of attention is really necessary, you can actually tire yourself out. Mental stamina is needed for labor as much as physical stamina, and both can become worn out if too much is asked of them. This means that at the first sign of a contraction, don't suddenly stop everything and focus on your breath with every contraction: "Oh, that's a contraction . . . focus, focus,

focus!" No, that will likely burn you out! Give the contractions only as much as they require and nothing more. Remember Chuck's line, "add nothing extra." Until contractions draw you in and demand that you focus to get through, let yourself do other things and be intentionally distracted away from labor. Even while deep in labor, giving your mind something to focus on other than the sensations pulsing through your body can be helpful. Some such purposeful distractions are music, labor projects, hiking, candle flames, photographs, art, or even movies.

Music

Let's talk playlists. One of the things I read all the time on my class intake forms under the question, "What are you already doing to prepare for labor?" is "Making playlists." Making playlists is becoming as common a childbirth preparation as having a baby shower. Here's the thing about playlists: the kind of music you *think* you'll want in labor now, before labor, might be entirely different from what you need when you're actually *in* labor. Most often, I hear expectant parents planning their playlists with calming music and music they love. While this can work, variety is needed.

One of my favorite stories about the power of music in labor is one I was not present for but heard from the mother herself. Rosie was giving birth at a birth center. She had lovely music on and labored a long time with limited progress. Her midwives told her that something needed to shift or they were likely going to have to transfer to the hospital to get some help to move labor along. Being deep, deep in labor, Rosie could only verbalize one key descriptive and complete word to let her team know what she needed: "Beyoncé!" With the change in music things shifted for Rosie's labor, and she was able to birth her baby at the birth center as she had hoped.

Remember too that sometimes what parents want in labor is silence, as even music can be too much for ears highly sensitized by labor.

Labor Projects

For some parents, labor might be slow to the point of boredom. It can be helpful to have a project in mind, something you might want to focus on when labor starts. Some parents cook and bake while in early labor while others clean, garden, or get creative with sewing, knitting, or something of that sort. Before having my first baby, I had planned a labor project expecting my labor to be long and slow like so many I had heard about. My husband and I had been married for about two years at that point and still hadn't put our wedding photos together into an album. I decided that I'd use early labor to finally do that. I bought the book and readied the photos for the time when they would be needed. Despite my best-laid plans, my labor started late at night and was quickly more than I could tolerate while assembling a wedding album! Sadly, my wedding photos are still in a bag waiting to be put into an album twenty years later. Oh well.

Still, in case your labor starts slowly as some do, think about what you might do to focus your mind while you navigate the early hours of labor. Might you enjoy baking, sewing, making art, or maybe something more physical?

Walking

Another great thing to do in early labor to help flow with the sensations *and* help with the positioning of your baby is to go for a hike or walk. I distinctly remember going to support a family in labor who were planning a home birth with a midwife I hadn't yet worked with before. I wore, as I always do to hospital births, my favorite Dansko clogs, as they are comfortable and stable, I can slip them on and off as needed, and I can wear them for hours on end if need be. I arrived at this labor at about midnight to the whole midwifery team, who had arrived a few minutes before me, getting everyone ready to go for a hike. And hike we did! We walked the Hollywood Hills for a few hours in the middle of the night. That was the last time I wore clogs to a home birth, especially with that team!

If you don't have beautiful natural spaces near you, just get out and walk around your neighborhood (assuming it's safe to do so). If the weather isn't conducive to going outdoors, walk around your home. If you have stairs, going up and down them can be helpful. I supported a family in labor during December when it was cold at night but lovely during the day. We walked during the day enjoying the winter sunshine, and when it got cold, we did laps around her one-room home until we left for the hospital where she planned to give birth.

Regardless of where you do it, walking rocks the pelvis and helps your baby move into a better position for birth. Remember, "motion is lotion."

Visual Distractions and Focal Points

There are distractions and there are things that actually help you focus more deeply. Watching movies and favorite shows is a popular early labor distraction for many parents. Some people like to go to a movie in a theater during labor, which can be a great labor outing so long as you are open to the very real possibility you won't see the whole film!

Some visuals can actually help you focus your attention when things get more intense. Watching the flickering of a candle flame is one such visual focal point. Real candles are not permitted at birth centers or hospitals due to the proximity to highly flammable items such as oxygen, which makes burning candles an at-home activity only. Battery-operated candles that kind of flicker can be taken to birth settings where real candles are forbidden. Remember that the sense of smell is heightened during labor, and unscented or barely scented candles are likely the only kinds you'll be able to comfortably tolerate.

 Try This

Practicing Ice "Contractions" with a Candle

Get the ice, towel or cloth diaper, and sixty-second timer you used in the ice practice as well as a candle and matches. Light the candle and let your attention focus gently on the flame. Pick up the ice and center your focus on the changing, shifting, movement of the flame. Come back to your outward breath. Return to the flame. When the timer goes off, put down the ice. How did you get through the ice contraction this time? What did you do that worked?

Other visuals can also be helpful. Before giving birth to our first baby, Brent and I created posters to support us during labor. We have kept them all these years, so I can share with you what was on each of them. Mine is a collage made of images and words cut out of magazines. At the center is a bouquet of mostly open stargazer lilies with the words "Be Present" directly under the flowers. There are also pictures of other flowers, new parents with their baby, labor positions, and lots of babies. There are words and phrases scattered around the board including "family," "you can," "stand-up and deliver," "inhale, exhale," "birth of a father," and "motherhood." During labor, the only part of this board I remember looking at was the central image of the lilies. So much so that when I was pregnant with my second baby, I made another board, but this time, the only image was a giant hand-drawn lily-like flower at the center with handwritten words all around the edges.

Brent's poster was very different from mine. At the center inside a green hand-drawn box he wrote the words "Selfless Support" and on either side of the box he wrote "Wife" and "Baby." Above the box he wrote, "Exhale • Tune in • Inhale" and below it, "This is not about you" (which was a note he wrote to himself to remember to turn his focus toward me). Down the left side of his poster was a list of phrases that we had found to be helpful when we practiced for labor prenatally. I don't remember seeing his board during labor, but I know it was nearby as I've seen it in pictures. What was surprising and especially noteworthy about Brent's board was how others benefited from it too. When my mom arrived after her all-night drive down from Northern California, she referenced the poster for what to say. She used the phrases on the board to support me while she held my hand through contractions and cooled my forehead between them. Without me knowing it, the board Brent made helped my mom seamlessly slide into a congruent supportive role even pretty late into labor.

Other great focal points you can use for visual support in labor are your labyrinth drawing from chapter 4; photos of beloved pets, family members, or inspirational places; fresh flowers, and art. There are some spectacular birth- and parenthood-related art pieces—paintings, etchings, statues, and more. Follow your interests and what inspires you as you collect and/or create visual supports for labor.

SACRED RITUAL ORDEALS

In today's birth culture, our willingness to view ordeals of any sort as capable of provoking meaningful change has all but vanished. The alchemists of the Middle Ages applied pressure and then turned up the heat in their attempts to turn lead into gold. While they might not have been able to actually transform basic items into gold, alchemical processes go far beyond the final product. Alchemy is the process of transmuting a substance of little value into something of importance. Even the baking of a cake is an alchemical process as it takes a gooey batter and by applying heat turns it into a fluffy and delectable dessert. So, too, can the challenges of labor, birth, and new parenthood be alchemical and transformative.

Taken personally, pain can be intolerable; it can feel as if it is about you rather than something that is happening to you. Being a victim of the pain in childbirth is very different from having pain as a part of childbirth, even when it is intense and overwhelming. Taken further into the landscape of ritual space, pain (as well as other forms of challenge) has a role as an alchemical fire—it is the fire upon which the metal of identity is forged. Pain is a common part of childbirth. Labor pain can be both purposeful in bringing about the birth of a baby and also productive in facilitating the birth of the parent. Pain in service of sacred transformation is sacred pain, although that does not necessarily make it any less painful! Pain can be an evil needing to be banished or a vehicle for profound change—and sometimes both simultaneously!

Receiving Pain Medicine

We must address the question of whether there are times when pain in labor is too much. In my experience as a parent and a professional, the answer is a clear yes. There are times in labor when the use of pain-relieving medication is warranted and compassionate, and the withholding of pain medicine is, or borders on, abusive. Even when pain is not so overwhelming as to be cruel, there are times when pain medications are needed or asked for by the birthing parent. I have witnessed parents for whom *asking* for pain medication was a flame far hotter and more difficult than enduring labor without it.

I have also witnessed times when an epidural was key to making a vaginal delivery possible. I remember a time when the resistance to the pain was actually working against the progress of labor and where receiving an epidural allowed the mother to relax and open as she could not do before, no matter how hard she tried.

Another time, I supported a mother with an early urge to push. When this happened, well before her cervix was fully dilated, the urge to push was extremely difficult to resist and as a result, her cervix began to swell from the added pressure inflicted by the unintended pushing. The epidural significantly reduced the urge to push and relaxed the mother, and those two things in conjunction, allowed her cervix to finish dilating.

Who can say what ordeals each person must face within the space of giving birth? What is true within the framework of birth as a transformative, initiatory process is that some form of challenge is the price of admission. Pain is an obvious version of an ordeal or challenge in childbirth, but it is definitely not the only possibility. Having an epidural to help with pain doesn't mean the initiatory ordeal of birth has been bypassed. Ordeal, to my mind, has far broader implications including missed expectations, anxiety, stress, fatigue, overwhelm, having to ask for help, and navigating the inherent uncertainty that comes with rites of passage.

Coping Scale

Most hospitals use a pain scale (see figure to the right) to assess how the pain is in labor. This is usually conveyed as a scale from zero (no pain) to ten (the worst pain you can imagine). This puts the focus on how bad it is rather than on how the parent is handling the intensity. Instead, try assessing how well you're navigating the pain and intensity on a different scale where zero means you're not coping at all, and ten means you're coping completely. This shift can help because it doesn't matter really how intense the pain is; what matters is how well you're coping and flowing with that intensity. This scale will give your team a better sense of how you are really doing.

PAIN, CONTROL, AND "LOSING IT" IN LABOR

For a culture driven by the prospect of control, the total alleviation of pain in labor is a highly attractive prospect. Pain can turn us into uncontrolled heaps of emotional expression, and, with today's medical advancements, being uncontrolled might be unnecessary. Images of control are highly valued, while loss of control, or wildness, is denigrated. Therefore, being able to maintain composure and a socially pleasing demeanor in the midst of labor is often desired to avoid being seen as "out of control." Here cultured Apollo conquers Artemis's wilderness.

The impulse to control the animalistic responses to pain in labor is not unique to pharmaceutical methods. Since the late 1990s, hypnosis for childbirth has become popular and useful for many birthing parents. It can be a powerful tool for parents working on connecting their mind and body, deepening their focus, and unhooking from unhelpful storylines that can spin in the mind when stressed.

My only concern about hypnosis for childbirth has to do with expectations. Parents who are only prepared with tools to make birth painless may find themselves ill-equipped to navigate the challenges if

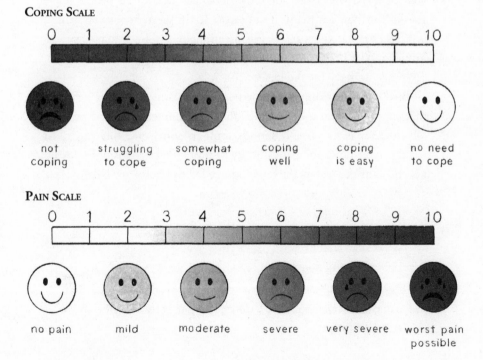

COPING SCALE

| 0 | 1 | 2 | 3 | 4 | 5 | 6 | 7 | 8 | 9 | 10 |

| not coping | struggling to cope | somewhat coping | coping well | coping is easy | no need to cope |

PAIN SCALE

| 0 | 1 | 2 | 3 | 4 | 5 | 6 | 7 | 8 | 9 | 10 |

| no pain | mild | moderate | severe | very severe | worst pain possible |

labor proves to be painful. Additionally, if the expectation is that by using self-hypnosis parents will remain calm and centered throughout, they may find themselves shutting off potentially helpful responses to labor such as making sounds and movement in an effort to appear calm and civilized. I believe in gathering supportive tools *and* speaking truth about the potential intensity, difficulties, challenges, and wild nature of labor.

Sometimes, people in labor *need* to "lose it," to let go of all socially appropriate behavior and become a heap of emotion—a raging beast or a puddle of tears. The wilderness of birth often invites such expressions. Just because outbursts of this type may not be wholly welcome in Apollonian society doesn't mean they aren't functional in the Artemisian wilderness of birth. Often, it is by letting go of ideas about "proper" behavior and instead moving as your body demands that opens the doorway of labor and allows it to flow forward toward birth.

Making Sounds

The sounds expressed during labor can make birth feel unfamiliar and wild to those who have not yet experienced it. Not all people make sounds in labor, but many, if not most, do. In Western cultures, sound is often denigrated because releasing animalistic sounds may create an impression of being "out of control," which goes against the godlike reverence we have for the idea of control.

But here's the thing: for some people, releasing sounds is *the* thing that supports them most during labor. Remember that your primary job in labor is to *open*. If sounds want to come out, but you resist letting them flow, energetically, are you opening or closing? Closing, which is antithetical to the opening needed to birth your baby.

Try This

Practicing Making Sounds

Make a high-pitched sound from your throat and head. Notice how that sound makes you feel. Do you feel clenched, tight, or fearful? Often high-pitched sounds elicit fear.

Now try dropping that sound down, low and deep, like the sound is coming from the bottom of your belly. Make it a low guttural sound that comes out with the exhale. What do you feel now? Do you feel tension or relaxation? What happens to your body when you make that lower-pitched sound?

Compare the two types of sounds in your mind. Which works better for helping you feel grounded, solid, and in your body rather than spinning in your mind? Usually the lower-pitched sounds help with letting go, whereas the high-pitched sounds feel tight and fearful.

Next, get a large bowl of ice or a bowl of ice mixed with water (Warning: this is actually more intense than just ice). Unlike with the ice contractions I had you do earlier, the intensity of the sensation from submerging your whole hand will continue *after* you remove your hand from the bowl. That means that this practice in some ways mimics more closely a contraction with a peak and descent.

Set your timer for thirty seconds and plunge your hand into the bowl of ice. Then find your exhale and let a sound come out with the breath. It may feel strange or forced at first. That's okay; keep going. You might have to fake it and make your exhale audible to begin to find which sounds help you. After the thirty seconds, rather than quickly drying and warming your hand, remove your hand from the bowl of ice but keep practicing. Once the sensation has subsided and you've had a chance to rest, try another few contractions like this, exploring how making sound can be helpful in letting go of tension.

When Cathlene was in active labor with her second child, her son came into the room with his birth buddy (his aunt) and [referring to his mother] said, "She is working *very* hard. And it's okay if she makes noises . . . that's what you do when you work hard." Their midwife told me that this simple statement from a toddler reminded the room of people and his mom that it was okay to acknowledge and vocally express hard work and pain.

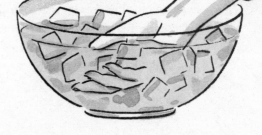

Some people like to use words instead of, or in addition to, more primal sounds. These might be supportive words, your baby's name, or, if you use them in your spiritual practice, prayers or mantras. Parents often find words that work for them in labor. My favorites are "ooopen" and "dooown" as they are not only a powerful reminder about what needs to happen, they are also well suited to the guttural nature of labor sounds.

Some parents may find that the words that want to flow out with sound and breath are curse words. If that happens for you, let 'em rip! It may seem strange, but it is often those for whom swear words are *not* a regular part of their daily life who find they have the most power. People like me who are serious potty-mouths may not find swear words very powerful, as we drop them at the slightest upset!

I invite you to *practice* making sounds prenatally for a few reasons. First, you might find through practice that releasing tension through the open expression of sound is actually really helpful in letting the flow of intensity wash over and around you. In that way making sound might help you navigate the intensity of labor. Reading about how making sounds might help is very different than trying it out for yourself in real life.

Additionally, practicing ahead of time will help familiarize you with the sounds possible in labor, and, if you invite them to participate with you, familiarize your partner too. Trying the sounds out prenatally can help reduce self-consciousness about making them during labor. It has been said that many pain medicines in labor are administered as much for the partner's comfort as for the one experiencing contractions. It can be very difficult to witness your loved one expressing pain, and the desire to do something to help can be overwhelming.

Fortunately, there is a lot that your partner can do to help you navigate the intensity of labor and support your emotional and physical journey through birth and into new parenthood. That's what the next chapter is all about.

Partners
on the Journey
to Birth

Partners deserve attention too and the couple is something entirely separate from the individuals who make it up. This chapter puts relationships in the center of our conversation about birth. Here's the other thing: individuals are transformed by birth and becoming a parent but so are relationships—often a lot!

Most aspects of this chapter are applicable to both romantic and platonic relationships. If you expect to have someone support you in labor or postpartum, be it a partner, husband, doula, friend, or family member, this chapter has tools to help improve the supported/supporter relationship for these unique situations.

THE GLORIFICATION OF INDEPENDENCE

One of the prominent ideals I see dominating Western culture is the glorification of independence—that idea that if you can do something by yourself, you should. This idealization of independence and self-reliance is deeply woven into the cultural mythology of the United States. We see the physical community changing drastically (from rural to urban to online) while extended family ties diminish. The media, with its images of the well-coiffed parents and successful entrepreneurs and celebrities, reinforces the idea of being successful on your own, with no mention of the team of people needed to create that appearance. We prefer the illusion of being amazing all by ourselves.

But this is not true. Everyone needs someone, especially parents. Flowing water is not a river without banks. We must break the idea that receiving help is a bad thing. Parenthood will likely teach you just how necessary it is to be well-skilled at asking for and receiving help. This chapter will teach you about both giving and receiving help now—before birth—as well as during birth and beyond.

THE RIVER: THE BANKS AND THE WATER

Labor, birth, and early postpartum are unique snapshots in time. During this phase of life, energy is heightened, vulnerability is often intensified, and many people find themselves in need of support and care they could never imagine wanting at other times of their lives. For parents, this is a time of such profound change that the bedrock of who they have known themselves to be can shake like an earthquake, with different Richter scale readings for each individual: some only sensing a small tremor and others experiencing major damage to the infrastructure of their lives. These feelings of instability are often caused by the shift from the earthbound energy of solidity to that of the ever-changing nature of water.

Imagine birth as a river, with its fluid watery existence, whether calmly moving forward, spinning in circles caught in an eddy, or stagnant and going nowhere. It may look calm on the surface while underneath, unseen, is a powerful force that is nearly unstoppable. Then there are the rapids. Rocks and narrow spaces make the water almost too powerful and dangerous to traverse. The water of the river is like the energy of birth and early postpartum. Stepping into labor requires the birthing parent to become the water with its changeability and its power.

For many modern people, this watery element is completely new, and its unpredictability can be destabilizing to well-ordered lives.

Many of us, myself included, are pretty used to the structure, order, and stability—the earthlike elements—of contemporary life. We feel comforted by what we can predict and measure with our lists, calendars, and planners, as well as the clock, which keeps us aware of the organizing principle of it all—time. The wateriness of birthing can upset this tried-and-true, well-ordered system. Even if it is the predictable energy we prefer, it is not the primary energy needed for birth.

In addition to the water, there is another part to every river—the banks. Without banks, rivers become swamps that go nowhere. The relationship between the water and the banks is a dynamic one: the water carves the banks, but the banks also contain the water. The banks hold and respond to the water—sometimes they are wide and spacious, giving the water lots of room to move or be still, while at other times they more firmly hold their ground. Even when the banks are made of solid rock, they are still responsive to the water—just look at the Grand Canyon for

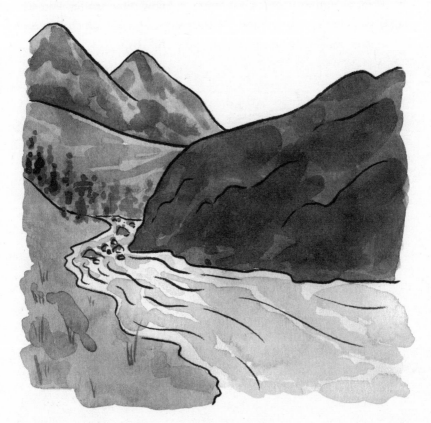

a brilliant example of how responsive rock can be to water. But the banks also direct the water and give it reliable support when it is intense and formidable. The dance between the water and the banks is powerful to behold in nature as well as in birth.

In labor, birth, and early postpartum, the birthing individual becomes the water. This often-unfamiliar elemental energy can be highly unsettling, especially if left without trustable banks to help hold it. The water of birth needs banks—trustable support that is both strong and responsive to the power of nature that can take over a birthing person's whole being.

The birthing person needs to step into the water for birth—to flow and change and roll with the unpredictable and sometimes chaotic nature of birth's course. To help you do this, you need people around you who can be your banks. You need to trust that no matter how intense or powerful the experience becomes, your support team will be there to support you. It's important to know those around you are solid and comfortable around the intensity of birth—much like the responsive and supportive banks of a powerful river.

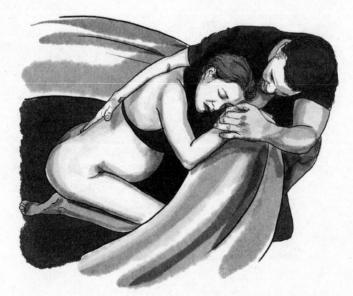

In some birth literature, being the banks to a laboring person's river is often referred to as "holding space." It's interesting that while in labor, many people say that they didn't *need* much from those around them; they only needed to know that what was happening and what they were doing was okay. Some of the most beloved midwives and obstetricians are notorious for a "hands off" approach where they don't get overly involved with what the laboring parent is doing unless needed. But they are doing something; they're holding space—simply being there, silently letting the parent know that all is fine. One of the reasons I believe doulas make a statistically significant difference in the birth satisfaction of their clients has to do with their ability to be reliable banks. They do this by holding space for whatever arises, maintaining a calm demeanor in the midst of situations that are unfamiliar to others, remaining unflappable to the raw expressions of labor, moderating their own big emotional responses, and rarely drawing attention to themselves.

This type of support isn't like the banks of the Los Angeles River where the natural banks have been fortified or even replaced by concrete, creating channels that lack flexibility. Concrete-like support isn't responsive and instead of holding space for the river, it forces the watery energy to conform to protocol, rules, or externally created norms. That type of energy in birth is rarely helpful. Births that are controlled by protocol or narrow ideas of "how all births should happen" are akin to concrete river banks. Each birth is unique and, therefore, even challenging births, like rivers attempting to carve through granite, still need responsiveness from the banks.

Directive, concrete, one-size-fits-all approaches are rarely effective, but neither is it helpful for a birthing person to be surrounded by people filled with their own emotional responses, whose shifting energy and opinions create instability. (Keep this in mind when inviting friends or family to be with you during labor.) That energy resembles the changing nature of water more than it does the reliable steady qualities of the banks. When there are no banks, the river is no longer a river; it's more like a swamp, where movement and direction are missing. Balance is needed between flowing water and responsive supportive banks.

The more a birthing person can trust the container holding them, the more easily they can flow openly into their birthing power. Both partners and birth companions can create a container that supports the birthing parent to rage, cry, soften, and melt by being reliable, stable, and present. This trust is cultivated with practice. You can begin that practice long before labor begins.

If a birthing parent is used to holding the banks in their daily life—containing and directing the energy of those around them—then stepping into the water of labor when the time comes can be very challenging. Often pregnant parents feel the pull toward the watery, less structured, more fluid parts of life whether they like it or not. Pregnant people label this shift as "pregnancy brain," referring to being forgetful, distractible, or fuzzy-brained. The pregnant brain begins to pull you into the water by making it harder to hold up the banks for everyone and everything around you.

Another way this pull shows up is within relationships. In moments of high stress, couples often polarize: one person takes on one energy while the other is naturally polarized to its opposite. Throughout pregnancy, the reality of becoming parents is often more noticeable and real for the parent whose body, mind, and life are already shifting profoundly as a result of the growing baby inside them. For the other partner, the reality might be slower to manifest. As the pregnant parent sees birth rapidly approaching, they often feel they need to let go of tasks, responsibilities, and items on their to-do lists. They know they can't maintain solid bank-like elements in their lives while also readying for labor, birth, and postpartum. I see this awareness express itself as antsiness and pressure to "get it all done." Partners often experience this as requests, sometimes to the point of nagging, to build the crib, paint the baby's room, install the car seat, or finally take all the classes needed in preparation for birth and postpartum.

How can the partner support the birthing parent to drop more fully into the role symbolized by the river's water? They can help by taking ownership of any of the things on the remaining to-do list. Encourage the pregnant parent to start letting go of being the banks in shared areas of your lives. For some couples, it works really well to step into this relationship polarity consciously and explicitly with one another, understanding the power of how these two energies work in response to each other. Often partners want to be the banks for their beloved during pregnancy, labor, and postpartum. This can be a powerful intention and one I have seen work really well.

Time and again, parents have shared how this allegory functioned as their main guide through labor. Partners often ask themselves, "How am I being the banks that my partner needs in this moment?" and birthing parents can ask, "How am I letting go into the flow of the water in this moment?" You do not need to intellectually know *everything* possible about labor and birth beforehand. Instead, understand the symbolic and elemental energy most functional for your particular role in labor and follow that as a guide to direct you. Imagery alone does not give parents everything that is needed for birth, but allegory along with the embodied knowledge learned through practice creates understanding and memory that is embedded more deeply than simply knowing something intellectually. This rooted knowing is often more retrievable than facts and figures during the rigor, fatigue, and excitement of labor.

LEARNING TO GIVE AND RECEIVE HELP

In one particular month, I worked with twenty-eight soon-to-be parents, each of them eager, excited, and somewhat fearful of the process before them. They arrived in my classes with the intention to learn about labor, birth, and how to best do it. Yes, they learned information about birth, but what they told me was most helpful and surprising was what they learned about themselves and their relationships to their partners.

One class I worked with was on their second of six weekly classes. We spent the first half of class processing the homework from the previous week. They were assigned a small amount of reading, but that wasn't the part of the homework of greatest interest. The partners were given the homework to do pain-coping practice two to three times between the two classes. It was their job to gather the ice, get a timer, set up the practice, and guide their beloved through the process. Birthing parents had a different assignment. They were asked to forget that their partner had been given an assignment at all. This is where it always gets most interesting.

Of course, it is nearly impossible for birthing parents to forget their partners' assignment, especially when they have been told to forget it. That is like saying, "Don't think of an elephant." All anyone can do after that is think of an elephant. But there are very specific intentions with these two different assignments.

Most pregnant people are the leading force on the quest toward parenthood, handling all the details of preparation. When it comes time for labor, the birthing parent generally wants their partner to magically be able to support them in just the way they want.

Most partners want to be engaged and helpful . . . they have the desire, but maybe not the tools. Practice gives partners the chance to figure out how to support, how to show up strongly, and how to become engaged in the process.

Pregnant parents, on the other hand, need practice *receiving* support. The primary intention behind this specific homework is to provide an opportunity to practice letting go of managing whether or not a particular birth-related experience or outcome happens. This gives the partner the opportunity to be the banks, and the birthing parent, the water. Used to being in charge of what happens regarding birth preparation and so familiar with being the driving force behind having everything ready in time, many birthing parents struggle between wanting to do the homework they have been given (to forget there is homework for their partner) and wanting to make sure they practice with the ice, which is the homework given to their partners. The value of this homework, which I only give in the first week, is to see what happens when the birthing individual lets go of directing and moves more fully into the metaphorical water, and the partner has the opportunity to step up and be the banks. Does it work? What is needed to make it easier for the birthing parent to step more fully into the river and the partner to more reliably hold the banks?

When processing the homework in classes, it is the experience behind what the couples did or did not do that is of greatest interest. As you explore working together as partners in new ways and in preparation for birth and co-parenting, explore what helps you both. What is it that each of you needs? Is more support needed in one direction or the other? What has been your dynamic in preparation for birth?

Has one of you done more of the heavy lifting toward readiness than the other? How has this balance or imbalance worked for each of you? There is not one right way to prepare. I offer up my understanding of birth and trends I've noticed from years of teaching classes, but it is up to you to determine what your relationship needs that is different from what is happening now. A great place to begin this exploration is by practicing supporting and being supported through ice contractions.

Building a Successful and Supportive Relationship for Labor

In my opinion, the main reason to practice with ice is not to prepare the birthing parent for contractions but to expose the couple to the experience of *supporting* and *being supported* while in an uncomfortable situation. This is rarely an intuitive skill. We are not used to being in a position of having to support our beloved while they navigate pain and intensity . . . and it's even harder when there are few things we can do to really help. Additionally, it is completely unfamiliar to most of us how to *receive* help from another when we are the one experiencing pain or discomfort. We need practice to develop these skills. Plus, it is better to try and flounder now when the stakes are low than to try in labor and have no idea what to do or what helps.

 Try This

Building Empathy

Let's add partner support to our ice contraction exercise from the previous chapter. Get some ice, a towel or cloth diaper, and a timer. Start with the partner holding the ice and the birthing parent offering physical support, verbal encouragement, or guidance. Do it for one minute—go!

Birthing parents, how was it supporting your partner? How did you know what to do and how to help? What did you notice you did or didn't do? Did it help your partner? How did you know if it did or didn't help them?

When I do the Building Empathy exercise in my classes, the birthing parents are usually quite blown away at how *hard* it is to be the support person. It is hard! It's hard to know what to do to help, to make a difference, and to really be supportive *in the way the other person needs*. You'll switch roles soon. For now, keep reading.

A Note for Birthing Parents

One of the purposes of these exercises is to help your partner grow their skills. Please keep this in mind as you begin to practice with partner support. They may not know exactly how to help the first time or second time or even a week from now. Give them the space to fumble, learn, try again, and ultimately develop the ability to help effectively. Remember, you're giving your partner the opportunity to try different forms of support so that they can develop a toolbox of skills for supporting your labor. In the process, you might be surprised by something you find helpful that you might never have thought of on your own. Build confidence *and* competence. The other purpose of these exercises is to give you the opportunity to practice opening to the *positive intention* your partner has to help. Let yourself *be supported*. This can take practice too! Soften into the gift of the love and focus behind their attempts to comfort you.

A Note for Partners

Supporting your beloved in the midst of the physically and emotionally intense experience of giving birth is likely unfamiliar and perhaps a bit daunting to you. Most of the parents I've worked with really want to be helpful and, if possible, make the intensity of labor a little less overwhelming for the person they love most in the world. Here's the thing: you do not need to know how to do it, how to be effective, or aim for perfection in order to *make a difference*. Showing up, holding space, being the banks of the ever-changing river of labor, while letting your beloved know how much you love them is often enough. And whatever happens, don't take it personally. If birth brings up intense physical sensations or emotions for your partner, you may well bear the brunt of their reactions to those experiences.

Keep in mind that the energy of birth will likely also be intense for *you*. You might need opportunities to take breaks, tend to your own emotions, eat, use the restroom, and maybe take a nap. Birth can be a quick sprint or a long, multiday marathon. Taking care of your well-being is important too. Here's why: At the end of labor and birth, there is this other, far longer experience that will likely require even more of your energy. It's called parenthood, and you will be needed when it comes. After what can be a draining experience of birth, the adrenaline rush subsides, and both parents are needed as life with a newborn sets in. Knowing that, be sure to get the support *you* need during labor. It is rarely possible for partners to be the banks during all of labor, especially if things take unexpected turns or there are particularly anxiety-producing events. This is one reason to hire a doula or ask a friend experienced in birth to support *both* of you during labor. It isn't just the birthing parent who needs help and support.

Even if you hire a doula or have someone else like a friend or a family member there to support you both, as the partner of the birthing parent, you offer something that no other person can: your love and awe for what your beloved is doing to birth your baby and the shared experience of having a baby together. These connections are uniquely yours. Others might be becoming grandparents or aunts, but only you share this special bond of becoming parents together. You two know each other in a very unique and profound way. This is your greatest strength in labor and in your support of your beloved. Share with them what you see, what moves you, the awe you experience watching them birth your baby, and the deep love you have for them. There is almost nothing as powerful to a laboring person than to hear that their partner is seeing them fully and loving them through it. This is powerful support. Use it and make memories in labor together.

General Support Suggestions for Labor

In addition to the unique support a beloved partner can offer, there are other universal skills and tips that can be useful to anyone supporting a person in labor. As you begin to practice with a support person during ice contractions, keep the following suggestions in mind. Discover what helps most. Take notes, try different things, and build your fluidity in this special dance.

- The most important thing you can do is watch the birthing parent and take your cues from what you observe.
  - » Are they managing the moment well on their own or do they need more support?
  - » Do they need something more or different?
  - » Where are they holding tension? Pay close attention to the key areas where birthing parents tend to clench: around the eyes/forehead, mouth/throat/jaw, shoulders, hands, and hips/buttocks.

- Be in rapport.
  - » If the birthing parent is quiet, internal, and still, don't come on like gangbusters with lots of words strung together without pauses like "OkayyougotthisKeepgoingBreatheRelaxGoodYougo." Doing this will take you totally out of rapport. Match the tempo and give space between your words so the birthing parent can incorporate what you've said.
  - » Similarly, if the birthing parent is moaning and groaning and breathing loudly and heading deeply into an animal place, don't bring out your ninety-year-old librarian voice with looong pauses between words. You'll lose connection this way too. Instead, try to match the energy, but a notch or two down on the intensity scale, just enough to stay in rapport *and* inspire inner softening around the intensity.

- Try using words laced with imagery or words that inspire visual as well as physical types of responses. Remember you want to invoke Artemis's realm rather than Apollo's, so nature-based imagery tends to be especially helpful. (Notice that these all end in "ing." Putting this ending on your support words changes them from sounding

like commands to feeling more like an invitation.)[1]
» Here are some of my favorite support words
and phrases: *softening, melting, opening,
floating, grounding, rolling over you, surfing the
wave, releasing, letting go, surrendering,* and
relaxing (use only in relation to a specific
body part that can actually be relaxed).

Use the words listed above along with what you observe, paying attention to those body parts mentioned in the list. For instance, if the birthing parent has their shoulders up to their ears (which is a pretty common response to the beginning of a contraction, as they try to brace against the downward feeling of opening that can be enormous), try saying something like "softening your shoulders as you exhale" or "surfing this breath . . . riding the exhale out." Don't worry about complete sentences. Laboring people actually like things short and simple as that resonates with their slower thoughts and more internal focus rather than activating their Apollonian mind with complex phrases and lengthy language-filled communications.

Keep in mind that as strong energy moves down and starts the process of opening, the body often wants to counteract those sensations by clenching against them. In other words, laboring people often tighten and close their buttocks and hips while also pulling their shoulders upward in direct response to the energy of opening and going down. What helps labor function is to support the energy of opening and dropping down. That's what you want in labor! You want the body to open and the baby to move down. If you see this upward, tight response, offer a suggestion for the opposite. Watch them and let what you see guide your support words.

Practice

Now that you have these general suggestions in mind, start putting them into practice so you can learn what works best in your relationship. What works for me to say to a client in labor is often very different from what their partner can say that feels natural to them. The only ways to find out what works are either to practice ahead of time or wing it in labor and hope something comes to you. I encourage practicing. It lays tracks of flow and receptivity in the brain and creates muscle memory for navigating difficult situations. This is one of the benefits of ritualized practice as well: it invites your brain to operate on autopilot. Well-established tracks are easier to access in the mental fog that often accompanies labor. So practice regularly!

Try This

Finding What Works

To practice together, start by having a brief conversation about what type of support you imagine will be helpful to you. Share ideas about words, types of touch, and even positions for support you imagine being helpful. Then get ice, a towel, and a sixty-second timer again as you did for the previous ice practice. Hold the ice in one hand, both hands, on the inner wrist, behind the ear, or some combination of these for one minute. During that time, the partner does what they can to support in the best way possible. When the timer goes off, put down the ice.

Giving Feedback

Giving and receiving feedback are important skills. This is the part of the ice practice that matters most in terms of building confidence and competence. These skills are not just important for practicing contractions but can be powerful abilities to have as partners in general. I encourage you to follow these guidelines.

Start by sharing with your partner what was helpful to you. Notice what worked . . . even if you have to dig deep to find something that was helpful, do it! Be specific. Let them know what they did or didn't do that worked for you.

This is not limited to giving feedback on the ice practice. In general, letting your partner know what worked first, before sharing how you want things to be different, works best for behavior change. The idea is that positive reinforcement for what works helps skills grow. If all we do is focus on what's not working or how they are failing, improvement will be slow or nonexistent. Since we want to grow skills for labor support, be sure to *focus on what's working.*

After you've shared what worked, then let them know one small thing they could do to support you even better. Rather than focusing on what didn't work, draw their attention to what they could do to *improve*. Your job as the one giving feedback is to help them build their skills and ability to support you. As the one receiving the support, paying attention to what is helpful also guides you to notice what's personally effective.

Two Simple Steps to Giving Feedback

1. Start with what worked, what was helpful, and what they did that was supportive.

2. Go to what they could do to make it even better and how they could improve their ability to support you in the ways you want and need.

Try This

Incorporating Feedback

Once you've shared feedback, do another ice contraction, switching hands and/or location of the ice. During this contraction, the partner incorporates the feedback they received and endeavors to improve their support skills. After the sixty seconds are over, again, put down the ice and give feedback in the same way as before—starting with what worked and moving on to improvements. If you have a clear instruction to give, such as "Don't touch my face," say it. In addition, try offering another option as well: "Don't touch my face. Try touching my shoulders or arms instead." Again, the idea here is to build skills and success. Part of that requires learning what to remove, but we also need to put tools into the toolbox. You can't do all jobs with a hammer, but if that's the only tool you have or know how to use, you'll likely try to use it with a screw, when a screwdriver would be much more effective! You need many tools so you can pull out the right one when needed. You will both benefit from a well-stocked and familiar toolbox!

Verbal Support

Often, birthing people tell their partners they like silence more than talking. This is great to know, but I've also seen many parents hit a point in labor where they need more than silence. Learning which words, phrases, and pacing are helpful is usually harder to master than silence. Practice with words, so you can explore ahead of time what's effective.

A typical action partners use to support is to ask the laboring parent a lot of questions during contractions. Remember that we want the birthing parent to drop into their Artemisian, animal, instinctual, and hormonally driven *body*. Questions put you in the head. They imply the need to answer. Questions take us up into the mind searching for a response. This moves the birthing parent out of their inner, nonsocial mode that is functional for labor and brings them out and up. Instead, encourage them to drop down and in. It isn't supportive to ask, "Do you like it when I touch your shoulders? How about your legs? Should I try something else? What do you want? Is this helpful? What else should I do?" and on and on. But if it isn't a good idea to ask a lot of questions, how then do you know if what you're doing in labor is helpful?

This can be puzzling. You are unlikely to get a string of supportive compliments: "Oh, sweetie, that's so great! I just love the way you're rubbing my back. You're truly the best! Thank you so much. You are so supportive!" Nope. Let me just tell you now, that is not gonna happen. The way you know if what you're doing is helpful is that you aren't told to stop. Yep, that's it. How's that for positive reinforcement?! If you aren't being told to do something else, either with a physical gesture moving you away or a verbal cue letting you know to do something different, then what you're doing is likely helpful. Sometimes partners find themselves deep in labor doing the same thing, saying the same words for hours on end. Just because you've become bored saying and doing the same thing, doesn't mean the one in Laborland has too. In reality, it is often the opposite. Repetition can be soothing for laboring parents and can help create a trance-like state that is supportive to the laboring mind. It is similar with repetitive touch; consistent reliable touch can give a laboring parent a sense of stability—banks in the midst of a turbulent river.

Partners, if you need a response regarding a question or you want to check in with your beloved about their needs, wait until the contraction has ended before asking. Remember that the hormonal trance of labor makes the brain move slowly. Keep your communication easy to respond to. Can you make the question one that can be answered with a yes or no or a shake of the head? If so, do that! Rather than asking if they're thirsty, offer a glass of water with a straw and invite them to take a drink. No conversation is needed, no discussion, no words at all. This is what you want. As much as possible, encourage the birthing parent to stay in an internal zone even when you're communicating. That zone is supporting the hormones to flow and labor to progress.

A note on humor: the first time couples practice with ice in my classes, there is always laughter and joking. For some couples, humor is an organic part of the language of their relationship. For those couples, humor can be an effective tool used successfully all the way through labor. Otherwise, humor only works until it doesn't. Keep in mind that humor, like questions, requires a response. Humor works best when there is an audience with whom to engage. This can bring a birthing person out of their inner zone in an effort to respond and laugh at the joke. So how do you know when humor no longer works in labor? You guessed it, the laughter stops. Again, watch your beloved. What you see will tell you a lot about what is and isn't needed in that moment, including humor.

Physical Support

Beyond verbal support, partners can offer physical support, and for many partners, this is the part they like best. Offering touch, massage, hip squeezes, bodily support for different positions . . . finally they get to *do* something that helps! Here are some suggestions:

Rhythmic Touch with Breath   Pay close attention to your beloved's breath. Watch it; then match your breath to theirs. With each inhale bring your hand up your beloved's back or arm. Then with the exhale, trace your hand down the other arm or the front of your beloved's body going over the belly and resting at the bottom of the belly but above the pubic area. What's important here is connecting the touch with the breath. It is not meant to be a strong touch; light, but not tickly is ideal. You want the birthing parent to feel the touch, but only so that it integrates and mirrors the breath.

Adding words that connect to the breath and the rhythmic touch can add another modality to deepen the focus. This does not have to be complex. You might say, "Drawing energy up your spine as you inhale. Softening as you exhale." Make your touch and your words connect with the breath. If your beloved needs help letting go and riding the intensity of the contractions, then a consistent, soft, downward stroke on the arms in rhythm with the exhale may be helpful.

Firm Massage Many laboring parents like firm massage on their backs, hips, shoulders, feet, or hands. Often the firm pressure from this sort of touch can counteract the intensity of the contractions. Many parents are surprised by just how firm they actually want the pressure. Try giving your partner a massage while they hold ice during a mock contraction. Find out what they like, where they like to be massaged, and what sort of pressure works best for them.

In labor, if you're looking for a way to support through a contraction, try massage. Have lotion or massage oil that is either unscented or only lightly scented available.

Counter Pressure Hip Squeeze As the pelvis stretches to accommodate a baby's head, laboring parents can feel pain in their hips and low back. Discomfort can also be due to a malpositioned baby. Regardless of the cause, a counter pressure hip squeeze can often offer some relief. There are a few different ways to use this support measure.

To do the double hip squeeze, have the pregnant parent on all fours, leaning on an exercise/birthing ball or supported by a bed or couch. The partner places the heels of their hands on the fleshy circles in the muscle of the buttocks below the hip bones (see figure below). You aren't pushing on any boney parts. With elbows out and fingers pointing upward, squeeze the buttocks toward one another and up toward the sky. This should feel good to the laboring parent. Practice this before labor to be sure you know what to do and get feedback ahead of time. Your partner should be able to guide you to make it feel better.

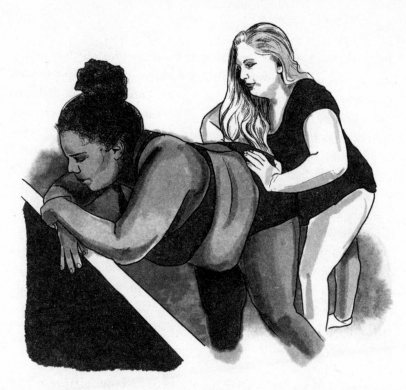

Another version of this doesn't require as much physical exertion on the partner's part. For this one, the birthing parent lies on their side on a firm but comfortable surface such as the floor, couch, or bed with their knees bent. The partner then finds that same fleshy part of the buttocks and pushes down and away from the body to mimic the action of squeezing together and up that you implemented in the version on all fours.

Partners, be warned that laboring parents often *love* this, which is great, but it can also be a very tiring form of physical support if implemented for hours on end. I remember using this with a dear friend in labor. She had some back labor (lots of sensation in the low back often caused by the baby entering the pelvis in a face-forward position, which can press the back of their skull onto their parent's sacrum). At some point in her labor, I tried the double hip squeeze and voila! She loved it! From that point on, she wanted it during every contraction. I probably did the double hip squeeze for close to ten hours! My arms were exhausted! I share this as a warning to not bring it out too early. The good news is, there are other options that give similar relief with less exertion.

Rebozo Another great tool in labor is the rebozo, which is a long, often sacred, piece of woven cloth used for several purposes and revered by people from many cultures, particularly Latin American. Rebozos can be utilized in many different ways in labor and offer a low-exertion alternative to the counter pressure hip squeeze. This is done by wrapping the rebozo (or a long scarf) around the hips and under the belly and tying it in back. Then a wooden spoon is inserted into the knot at the sacrum and twisted until the right pressure is reached for the pregnant parent. Using the rebozo in this way provides the birthing parent some counter-pressure relief on their own.

This is only one valuable way to use this amazing, traditional tool; there are many others. I think rebozos are truly wonderful, and I recommend learning more about using them from a trained source. You can ask your doula to show you how to use one (if they've been properly trained to do so), and there are also in-person and online classes that demonstrate proper use.[2]

Support Positions It can be helpful for you and your partner to have some familiarity around positions that might be supportive during labor. I'll include a few here, and there are many images and charts available online that can work as a good reference during labor when you're wondering what else to try. You can download one I like from my website at brittabushnell.com/labor-positions.

Try sitting behind your partner so they can rest against your chest. Have something supportive behind you such as a wall or the headboard of a bed so that you don't exert yourself unnecessarily. Another option is to stand against a solid wall with your back completely touching the wall without hunching. Place your feet at least hip distance apart and keep your knees slightly bent. Let your beloved lean against you and support them under their arms with your arms at right angles. Your beloved might want to drop into a little bit of a squat during a contraction and need your support. Holding some of their weight during a contraction can be challenging and makes it critical to be well supported by the wall and the position of your body. Don't muscle through. Be sure to take care of your body's needs as well.

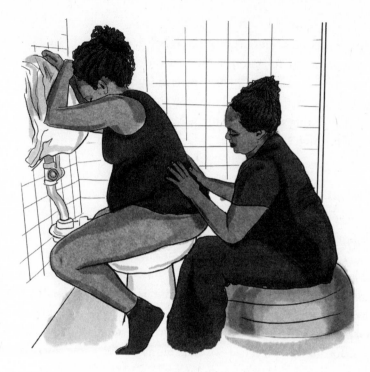

Sitting backward on a toilet seat with a pillow on the tank for resting your head is a favorite position for laboring parents because it leaves your back available for touch or massage (see figure below). Remember that bathrooms tend to be favorite labor locations, and this position tends to help parents to relax their pelvic floor since doing so is something we've done for years while using the toilet. This position can be mimicked by sitting on a birthing ball (which allows for movement) while also leaning on an elevated bed (which makes it a good option when staying close to a fetal monitor is necessary).

Connection

If you remember anything from this chapter, I hope it's that connection as a couple is one of the best and most supportive elements during labor, birth, and beyond. Only the two of you are becoming parents the day your baby is born. One way or another, your love has helped bring this baby into being. The love and connection between you is profoundly powerful for labor and birth. No one else in the room is also having a baby. This bond is uniquely yours. Honor that. Use it. Loving support from a partner is difficult to substitute. Partners do not need to be fully versed in all things birth or be experts at labor support. What partners provide is something entirely special and profoundly important. Tap into that during birth. Ride the waves of labor together. Share in the awe of birthing your baby.

About Doulas

On that same trip to India I mentioned in the previous chapter, one of the places my travel partner, Tora, and I explored was Nepal. I was eager to go trekking in the Himalayas as some good friends of mine had done so, and their stories were pure magic! Tora's mother, Denise, was also eager to do a trek, and so she met up with us in Kathmandu. The two of them were insistent about hiring a guide and porters. I was resistant and, as a prolific backpacker, unwilling to hire a porter. Five of us embarked on a three-week trek called the Annapurna Circuit—the three of us, a hired guide, and a porter for their packs.

That experience taught me more than I could have imagined, especially about my former "go it alone" mentality. Having our guide, Agasta, was the single best decision I didn't make on that trek! Sure, I had read books about trekking in general and about the Annapurna Circuit in particular; I had a map, a phrase book, and all the equipment I might need. But it was Agasta, with his experience and knowledge of the area, villages, language, people, and customs that made the experience truly extraordinary. He was the one who guided us over the Thorong La Pass at almost 18,000 feet in the dark and on freshly fallen snow, a journey that to this day is still one of the most spiritual experiences of my life. And, when I got sick about halfway through the trek, it was Agasta who found a spot for us to stay between villages and hired a shaman with two thumbs on each hand to conduct an unforgettable healing ritual for me. No guidebook could have created the magnificence of those two experiences no matter how closely I had read it. That trek was truly life changing, due in part to having an experienced and knowledgeable guide.

Couples often wonder if they should hire a doula. Maybe your friends had wonderful births and didn't hire a doula, why should you? All I can say is that doulas are like guides for the trek of labor. They know the landscape, are familiar with the people, sights, and sounds, and know special tricks that just might help you over a peak or through a valley or help facilitate that magical experience that lands firmly in your memory forever. And doulas are there for the whole family. They support partners, too, helping them understand what's going on, get food, rest, and much needed breaks, and they can also guide partners in better ways to support the laboring parent. You do not have to go it alone. There are others who have trekked before you and know the terrain. Ask them for help.

Friends or Family in Place of a Doula

Even when they know the value of a doula, not all families are able to hire one, and some parents prefer to labor on their own without help. Although I had that wonderful experience trekking with a guide and knew about doulas, I did not choose to hire one for either of my births! However, I knew I would want support in labor and asked my mom to be there to help me. Fortunately, she had supported several friends and extended family members in labor before, and I felt comfortable sharing my labor journeys with her. So while I didn't have a professional doula with me in labor, my mom did have some labor support experience that I was able to rely upon. As with all things related to birth and parenthood, you have to decide for yourself what feels right for you and your family.

8

Someone's Parent

Today's culture reveres innocence. Culturally speaking, we prefer to stay in the fantasy that we are innocent rather than own personal or collective responsibility. We would rather protect our innocent beliefs than speak truthfully about the state of the world, injustice, or the realities of life and death. We take an "I didn't know" or "It wasn't me" approach to difficulties, claiming innocence and eschewing responsibility. Evidence of this cultural ideal can be seen in political debate, in the way horrible parts of our history are ignored or silenced, in the thousand different ways we judge others (especially those less fortunate), and in submission to the idea that "that's just the way things are; you can't change them."

Innocence is understandable in children, but not in adults. Children need their parents to be adults and not just older children. That doesn't mean we lose the ability to play, but rather that we know how to face difficulty when it arises with resilience and flexibility, that we take responsibility for our actions, and that we are open to hard realities and don't hide in idealism and wishful thinking. Kids need us to model these behaviors so that one day they, too, can be resourceful, self-responsible, and capable adults. We need to *become* adults so that we can ultimately *raise* adults.

BECOMING A PARENT

Becoming a parent for the first time involves turning the archetypal wheel of families—the child becomes the parent, and the parent becomes the grandparent, and a new person enters the family as the child. Shifting from the child to the parent requires a certain amount of maturation. It is a substantial and sometimes tricky change. When you become someone's parent, you take on responsibility for your child. No longer are you the child to be guided and directed by your own parents. Now *you* are the parent! As such, begin trying on the mantle of parenthood during pregnancy. Some ways are fun; some are harder.

Rehearsing

Before you have a child, begin exploring how you would like to be as a parent. Read books, babysit for a friend or family member, or discuss parenting styles you see within your community or on TV with your partner. If you have no experience with babies, I recommend that you take a newborn care class prenatally as a way to bring to the forefront of your awareness that a *baby* is on the other side of pregnancy. Preparing for parenthood can also include exploring your options for postpartum and beyond (we'll discuss these more in chapter 11).

In addition to the ideas listed above, start being a parent to your baby in utero. Talk to them, sing to them, read stories, or play music just for them. Many parents do this instinctually, but the act of doing so is more than just an impulse; it is a way to begin rewiring your brain for being *someone's parent*.

One of my favorite rituals during my pregnancies was to sing lullabies at bedtime and in the bath. Singing to my unborn child each night after a long day brought the reality of becoming a parent to my consciousness. This ritual may seem insignificant to some, but it was profound in its simplicity. It had added benefits after birth too. Hearing develops about halfway through pregnancy, so by the time your baby is born, it already knows your voice.

Find a lullaby or two that you enjoy singing to your baby. Don't worry about your voice; your baby loves how you sound! Remember that the songs you sing don't have to be traditional lullabies. I know many parents who have sung Beatles and Coldplay songs. Sing what you love! You might be singing it every night for years to come!

What are other ways to incorporate parenting practices into your life with your baby even while they are still inside you? Find or make ways to experience the role of parent now. One of the most important ways to do this is in advocating for yourself and your child with health-care professionals.

Advocating for Yourself and Your Child

As a parent, you take on the role of primary advocate for your child. This role is one you will hold until they can advocate for themselves. Early in pregnancy, you begin the role of advocating on your child's behalf in discussions with your health-care team, negotiating with your employer regarding parental leave, dealing with insurance issues, and in conversations with loved ones regarding baby showers, appropriate gifts, baby names, and more! Learning how to advocate strongly for your growing family is a key skill in the process of maturing into parenthood.

Consent and Refusal

There is a lot of discussion and press these days about consent and refusal in general as well as around medical issues. These conversations around birth address the right to be informed before making a decision to consent to or refuse/decline a procedure. (I use both *refuse* and *decline* as there are times you might have to be forceful and refuse, while other times it is sufficient to simply decline without added intensity. Pick the word that works best for you and the situation.) The tools I share in the next sections will help you get the information you need to be informed enough to make decisions about your health care.

But what exactly is informed consent, and why is it important? The generally agreed upon definition of informed consent is "the willing acceptance of a medical intervention by a patient after adequate disclosure by the physician of the nature of the intervention, its risks and benefits, and its alternatives with their risks and benefits."[1] While that might seem like a mouthful, most important in that definition is the phrase "willing acceptance." In many places you are legally and ethically entitled to decision-making autonomy regarding your care.

One of the confusing areas regards the consent forms often signed upon arrival at the hospital or as part of your contract for care with a midwife. ACOG differentiates informed consent from the *consent form*. They affirm that informed consent is agreement to the proposed care *following* a discussion regarding "the nature of the intervention with its risks and benefits and of the alternatives with their risks and benefits." Whereas, "the consent form only documents the process and the patient decision. The primary purpose of the consent process is to protect patient autonomy."[2] Therefore, according to the governing body for obstetricians and gynecologists, parents are entitled to active involvement in the decision-making process, including final say.

Sadly, this is not always practiced in regard to pregnancy care, and several gray areas exist. Maturing into parenthood includes learning about your rights and understanding what is, and is not, consent where you live. Additionally, while aggressively standing up for your choices might be your right (depending on where you live), alienating your care team when you need them doesn't always work in your favor.

Building a Bridge

It can be hard to remember that the professionals supporting you through pregnancy and birth work for *you*—you hired them! Hopefully you've decided to work with them because you believe they have the best intentions for your well-being. If you don't think this is true, or their strategies of care don't align with yours, then find someone else if you are able. I like to believe that the medical team supporting any family I work with has the best intentions for the family. Everyone has bad days, certainly, but I believe people are drawn to work with birthing families because they want to help.

Medical professionals know a lot about birth and being asked questions can sometimes put them on the defensive. It shouldn't be your job to have to smooth the feelings of those you have hired to help you, but in reality, we have to do so frequently, and not just in labor. Pregnancy is just the beginning of a long career of advocating on behalf of your child's well-being, be it with teachers, coaches, or pediatricians. The opportunities will be numerous for years to come!

When two or more people come together to affect a course of action, they often do so with strategies in mind. Conflict arises when two strategies clash, or when either party believes they know best. When people begin strategic discussions on the battlefield, they are bound to have stressful conflicts.

Additionally, when you clash with your providers and become defensive, are you energetically opening or closing? Closing. And the number one thing that needs to happen in labor is opening. It is difficult to be both offense and defense at the same time. You need to find ways to stay open while still advocating for your wants and needs. Building a bridge with your provider is a way to do that.[3]

Instead of clashing and hitting a wall of disagreement over strategy, start by building a bridge between you and your provider. This process involves actively listening for the concern and the positive intention behind what is being suggested. This can be unfamiliar and clumsy but usually gets better with practice. Let me share an example.

A health-care provider sees that labor has been going on for a long time with little progress. Upon assessing the situation, they suggest breaking the bag of waters to help speed things along. You might know that labor can take a long time and progress sometimes stalls, especially prior to six-centimeter dilation. Your impulse might be to respond with some form of "No, I don't want to do that." While this is completely within your rights, you might have more success building a bridge of understanding and partnership with your provider by starting the dialogue in a different way. Try this instead:

- Listen for the concern (labor going on too long).

- Listen for the positive intention (to help get things going).

- Voice what you hear.

In this example, that might sound something like, "Okay, so you think this is going on too long and you'd like to get things going. Is that correct?" By voicing clearly that you have heard both their concern and their desire to be helpful, they are far more likely to stay connected and supportive rather than becoming defensive. When providers are more engaged and less defensive, they are more likely to work as part of your team than act as the all-knowing dictator against whom you have to fight to get your way. Practice building a bridge as often as you can in your life now, before giving birth. Try it in appointments with your prenatal care provider, when interviewing pediatricians, nannies, doulas, with extended family, or even at work with your coworkers. From my experience, it's magical!

Informed Decision-Making

Getting good information during labor isn't always easy. It can be helpful to have your labor partner learn how to build bridges and ask good questions if you find you need help. Engaging with your team personally can sometimes be challenging from within the hazy fog induced by labor hormones. Having someone else ask the questions removes much of the work of acquiring necessary information, which allows you to hear the answers given and make decisions based on what you hear. This way birthing parents remain receptive, retaining connection to their more internal state rather than having to become overly engaged intellectually. I encourage you to share bridge building and the next process with those sharing in your birth journey.

Once you or your labor partner have built a bridge of shared positive intention, then ask the questions that will get the information needed to make an informed decision for yourself and your baby. I don't remember where I learned this acronym, as it was so long ago, but I still love it and use it with my students, although I've changed it a bit over the years.

B.R.A.I.N.

B–Benefits   How might (the proposed course of action) be helpful?

R–Risks   When what you propose doesn't work, what happens? What are some of the unexpected side effects that can happen with this, even if rare? When you've seen this procedure go poorly, what has happened? Under what situations is doing (what is proposed) not a good idea? Are there other procedures that go along with this one that might be helpful to know about (e.g., catheter, IV fluids, and continuous fetal monitoring with an epidural)?

A–Alternatives   Is there anything else we could try? What are some other things you've tried in similar situations that have been helpful? Have you seen or heard of other things we might try first?

I–Intuition   How do I think/feel about this? What is my intuition saying is the next best action or inaction to take? (Keep in mind that it will likely be your partner or another labor companion asking these questions. If this is the case, be sure to tell them what you think of the proposed suggestion.)

N–Not yet   What if we wait an hour (or thirty minutes—base the amount of time on the situation)? This question helps you quickly assess the urgency of the situation. If you ask, "What if we wait an hour?" you will learn very quickly if the situation is perilous and action is necessary now for the health and safety of either parent or baby.

You do not have to ask all of these questions or ask them in order. I like to start with "What if we wait an hour?" This question gets you powerful information quickly. You learn how urgent the situation is from the perspective of your care provider. Next, I suggest asking about alternatives so you can understand the options, followed by benefits and risks.

Then pause, ask for time to discuss or ponder the situation alone if you need to, and check in with yourself and your partner about how *you* feel about the proposed action. Laying that out in order would spell N.A.B.R.I.—not nearly as memorable, but from my perspective, more effective!

One of the great benefits of walking through these steps—building a bridge and then asking good questions—is the ability to slow down the decision-making process. Remember that in labor the mind moves slowly. As such, many parents find that keeping up with conversations had with people not in labor (including health-care providers) adds stress. It is common for parents to feel they were pressured into taking an action in labor that they later regretted. When situations are not imminently dangerous, slowing things down often helps everyone feel better about whatever decisions are made.

What's on the Menu?

Most parents come to a point in pregnancy where they have learned enough about labor and birth to know, more or less, how they would like their birthing experience to unfold. Like them, you have probably chosen your provider, selected your intended birth location, and explored different options for managing the pain and intensity of contractions. Hopefully, your provider and location are well matched to support you in the way you desire. You are unlikely to have a birth that is minimally managed if your provider and/or location don't offer that type of birth on their regular menu. You won't get good Thai food at an Italian restaurant. If you want a water birth, but your provider works in a location that has no tubs, you aren't going to have a water birth. If you want the option of using an epidural, home and birth center midwives are not going to be able to provide that without transferring care to a hospital-based provider. If you want to go into labor spontaneously, but your doctor has a very high induction rate, your odds of getting the birth you want are low. In fact, recent research by Neel Shah, an assistant professor of obstetrics and gynecology at Harvard Medical School, found that the number one risk factor for a cesarean birth is which hospital a parent uses for delivery.[4]

If your provider and intended location don't regularly provide the type of birth experience you desire, you aren't likely to get what you envision for your birth. Or you might have to do what my Mexican-food-loving kids did while we were in India and make naan and dal "burritos" at every meal. They found a way to make what *was* on the menu resemble what they wanted, but it never fully satisfied their desire for a true California-style burrito. Find out what's on the "menu" with your provider and at your intended birth location. It's important to understand that if you're ordering something that isn't on the usual menu, you are likely going to be making it up from what's already there or getting something that *is* on the menu, whether you're hungry for it or not.

Keep in mind that even when your hopes for your birth are on the usual menu of care at your intended birth location and with your selected care provider, labor, birth, and parenthood are not a restaurant where you can simply order up your desired outcome. Making sure your desires are well matched betters your odds but doesn't provide certainty. Even if something is on the menu, it doesn't mean it will be available to you the day you hope to order it. As with all things birth-related, develop resilience and strength so that you can respond to the events of labor as they unfold in the moment.

FACING FEAR

In a culture that values light, reason, and social graces, Artemisian values are often vilified, making the initiatory process into parenthood ever more challenging. We are often removed from the transformative energy that lies within the great mystery, darkness, and creative chaos of hardship.

Beyond stepping into the role of parent with all that implies, awaking from innocence and moving toward true maturity involves preparing for the *challenges* as well as the *joys* of new parenthood. The maturation process available through childbirth involves the possibility of pain, failed expectations, great difficulty, and depths of despair.

It is common in many birth circles to minimize and soften the potential difficulties of giving birth. Well-meaning friends and professionals talk of orgasmic and painless births. They change "scary" words like *contractions* and *pain* to words like *waves*, *rushes*, and *intensity*, and even offer impossible promises like, "That won't happen to you." Shielding new parents from potential challenges maintains their innocence and naiveté. When that innocence is lost—as it is bound to be at some point—and parents are required to face difficult challenges in childbirth or parenthood, they can become paralyzed, victimized, or otherwise emotionally wounded. By avoiding potentially challenging truths, well-meaning guides actually reinforce fragility rather than inspire true strength.

In her book, *Healing Through the Dark Emotions*, psychotherapist Miriam Greenspan helps to explain this impulse.

When an innocent child looks directly into your eyes and asks you to explain evil, natural catastrophe, and human vulnerability, there is nothing more compelling than wanting to reassure her. We want to say: You are perfectly safe. There is no danger to you. You will not be kidnapped, killed, or hurt. You will not die by earthquake, flood, tornado, or fire. We will take care of you and protect you. Nothing bad will ever happen to you. The bad things only happen to other people. Far away. Not here. Not you. Ever.

These answers, we know even as we speak them, are lies. The white lies we tell for a good cause: to reassure a frightened child. They are the reassuring illusions that deny the truth of human vulnerability. And as any parent knows, we spin them for ourselves at least as much as for our children. Of course somewhere we know that we are teaching our children the illusion of invulnerability. Of course we know that there is never an absolute guarantee of safety for any child or any adult, that we cannot shield them or ourselves from unexpected harm. But we try to shield them from the fear of harm. Often, we end up teaching them how to be afraid of fear, and afraid of vulnerability, rather than how to know that fear and vulnerability are part of every life and how to cope with them.[5]

The impulse to protect the vulnerable from images of difficulty and evil is a cultural phenomenon not unique to birth. Throughout most cultures, images of darkness and difficulty are minimized and even eliminated in order to shelter those we believe to be innocents.

I believe in speaking truth rather than fantasy. I believe in your ability to face even difficult challenges with resilience, strength, and maturity.

Speaking the whole truth about birth means discussing those things you think won't apply to you as well as the less glamorous aspects of labor and birth, including fear. Sometimes, *fear* is too strong a word to describe the feelings parents have facing the unknown. Perhaps you just have concerns or things you're hoping won't happen. If your level of worry is nothing larger than a slight concern or as big as a full-blown terror, there are things you can do to help relieve some of the stress that hitchhikes on the back of pregnancy worry.

Unexpected things happen in birth just like they do in life. The unknown is an intrinsic part of the unfamiliar landscape of birth and new parenthood. And some fears can be lessened by becoming more familiar with the aspects of the feared experience. Gather courage. Learn more about what you fear. Research. Ask questions. Get curious. Be bold. You gain strength not by pretending your fears don't exist but by looking them in the eye.

Let's take an unwanted cesarean as an example. Most people reading this book are likely hoping *not* to have a cesarean delivery. Many parents go to great lengths to avoid a surgical birth. Still, about one in three babies born in the United States is born surgically, so addressing this fear is an important one. I will address cesarean births directly in chapter 10. For our purposes here, I want to address the *fear* of a cesarean rather than the cesarean itself.

In the face of a fear, ask yourself, "What steps need to be taken *now* to reduce the possibility that a cesarean (or whatever you fear) becomes part of my birth?" Answers to this question might include things like asking your provider more questions about the situations in which they feel a cesarean is needed, exploring with your provider what happens if a cesarean becomes necessary, or finding out the cesarean rate for your provider and intended birth location.

Addressing risk factors is important and a pretty common preparatory tool utilized by parents on the threshold of birth. But we have to take it further than reducing our chances of unwished-for situations. Once you've explored aspects of the unwished-for situation that can be addressed ahead of time and mitigated the chances of it happening in the first place, then it is time to face your fear head on.

Gather your courage and ask this question: "*If* this were to become part of my birth, what would I need to know or do to keep going?" Let yourself imagine having to face your unwished-for event. Invite your mind to picture it happening. Without changing the situation or magically having it remedied, dive in to the image of the situation you hope won't happen. Picture yourself doing the best you can in the face of it. Imagine that you are receiving the support of the most nurturing part of yourself—that part of you that is not only wise but also loving regardless of what's happening. Imagine that nurturing, wise, loving part whispering in your ear as you navigate this unwished-for event. What does that inner voice say to you? How does that wisest and kindest part help and guide you?

This kind inner voice isn't judgmental. It doesn't blame or shame; nor does it puff you up with the empty promises of a cheerleader. It doesn't sound like, "You suck" or "You're the best!" Instead, it offers the tenderness of a loving and wise parent speaking to a hurt child. "You wish it were different and you're sad. I am here. Even though this happened, you are okay." This special voice speaks to the part of you that is consistent and unflappable even when the shit's hitting the fan! When you've found this voice, it can be surprisingly low key. Judgmental voices often dress up in cheerleading outfits and scream at you to feel something you aren't actually feeling. You've likely experienced this at some point when you've felt down about your abilities, success, or progress, and someone (or your own inner voice) says, "Don't worry, you're the *best*!" While this sort of empty accolade can be nice to hear, it rarely tends to our vulnerable heart, and the suffering often continues. That's because those sorts of statements unconsciously tell you that what you *are* feeling isn't okay and that you *should* be feeling something else instead. Dark emotions such as grief, fear, anger, and shame are not consoled by affirmations. Emotions of this type need space to be felt, to be okay, to be held just as they are without rejection or denial. Awakening the parent within us includes acceptance for these tough and stigmatized emotions.

When you're ready, loop in partners, parents, your doula if you have one, or anyone you plan to have support you. Keep in mind that the objective of discussing fears is not to have others brush them aside or rescue you from them. Instead, focus on what they can do to help you if this unwished-for situation were to occur: "If this *were* to happen, please help me with _____ " or "Thank you for helping reduce the probability of this happening, and would you also help me brainstorm what you and I could do to help make it a better situation in the event it actually were to happen?" Keep the focus on engaging coping skills and gathering strategies for resilience rather than promises and reassurance.

Exploring these questions may not alleviate your fears, but they will help you better navigate unwanted events. If you have fears that spin regularly in your mind, often unbidden, address each of them in this way. Remember that becoming fearless is not the goal. You want to be self-caring and resourceful while you are feeling your fears.

What Happens in the Cocoon

Birth transforms an individual into a parent; one identity dies, and another is born. It is often said that the opposite of death is life. Really, life is what happens *between* birth and death. Birth and death are the bookends of life, and as such, stand in a somewhat awkward partnership of which most of us are unaware. In the West where denial of death is the cultural norm, it can feel not just uncomfortable to think about death in relation to childbirth but also as if something is *wrong* with us if we do.

But a butterfly does not grow wings without dying to its caterpillar self. Inside the cocoon, the caterpillar is reduced to goo. While the nervous system remains, the structure of the caterpillar—that which makes the caterpillar recognizable as a caterpillar—dissolves. This occurs unseen by the outside world, hidden inside the chrysalis. Then slowly, over time and with a certain amount of magic, that goo begins to reform into something new that has never existed before. The caterpillar morphs into a creature with wings and antennae. It becomes something full of color and gifted with new abilities like the capacity to fly! This is no small feat of nature. Still, this transfiguration is not possible without the death of the caterpillar to its life *as a caterpillar*.

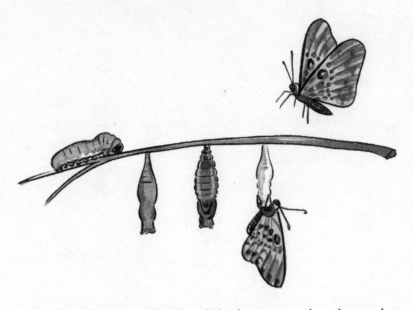

However intertwined birth and death are in myth and metaphor, in contemporary culture, there may not be a more slippery slope to traverse than to invite death into any conversation about birth.

DENIAL OF DEATH

The further we move away from an agricultural life on the farm where birth and death are normal parts of life, the more anxious and death-denying we become. As the gods of science and technology advance, so, too, does the promise of immortality.

The West continues to deepen its denial of death. The elderly are no longer viewed as an important part of society from whom wisdom flows. Instead, they are put in homes and separated from society. Doing so protects the rest of us from witnessing the truth of old age, sickness, and death, which in turn, allows us to continue in the unconscious fantasy that we might be able to avoid those realities of being human.

There is hope in all areas of life that people can improve, even escape, the limitations of our bodies, not through faith in the everlasting life promised by most religions but through better information, more modern technology, and ever-expanding progress. Science has become godly. Perhaps in no place is this connection more obvious than in the hospital labor room.

Death and Childbirth

One of the universal fears in childbirth is the fear of death. It's no wonder this subliminal fear is so prevalent. As recently as about a hundred years ago, "for every 1000 live births, six to nine women in the United States died of pregnancy-related complications" and one in ten babies did not live to their first birthday.[1] We have been wired over millions of years of evolution to be afraid of this outcome, even though it is uncommon today. During my years working with soon-to-be parents, I have watched the faces, read the body language, and navigated the emotional minefield that bringing up this topic creates. Still, the conversation around death in regard to birth is essential.

It is important to remark here that birth and death are not only a symbolic pair. On occasion in birth, death can be very real. Babies and birthing parents still die or nearly die in childbirth. Birth is not without risks, but the risks aren't equal for all people. Black babies are at double the risk of death compared to white babies, and black birthing parents are about three times as likely to die in childbirth as their white counterparts.[2] Inequity in birth is significant and predominately due to systemic racism, as well as access to care and classism. White, rich, urban people have the best outcomes. The statistics for those who are poor, rural, and/or black are inexcusable and must be dramatically improved.

While mortality rates have dropped significantly in the past hundred years, they are still high enough that almost every birthing parent knows of someone who has either lost a baby in birth or knows of a person who died (or nearly died) in the process of giving birth. While people are far more likely to survive childbirth today than just about any time in history, birth is not without risk.

Additionally, many parents come in contact with death in the process of getting pregnant. Few people feel they can openly talk about the loss of a pregnancy—wanted or otherwise—among friends or family. Pregnancy loss is a modern-day unspeakable. For families who have faced pregnancy loss, death is not only symbolic but very real.

A birthing parent faces the inner death of their previous identity on the journey into birth and their new identity as a parent. It is important to note that in all human transitions, rebirth is only possible through some form of death of the old identity. Without an innate understanding of this interconnected relationship between birth and death, modern people caught in a culturally enabled yet subconscious denial of death may prevent the possibility of the spiritual and psychological rebirth available to them as they become a parent.

JOURNEY TO THE UNDERWORLD

Perhaps my favorite tool for learning to embrace the unexpected has been the Sumerian myth, *The Descent of Inanna*. This story tells of the journey of Inanna, the Sumerian Queen of Heaven and Earth, as she descends to the Underworld to visit her sister, Ereshkigal. Okay, I don't blame you if you furrow your brow at these unfamiliar names and ponder, "What in the world do these characters have to do with my birth?" It's hard to fathom how an ancient myth from a faraway land might be useful in preparation for childbirth. Let me assure you that I have shared this story with parents in my childbirth classes for well over a decade and parents often speak to it being one of the most profound parts of our time together. In many cases, the myth of Inanna is the most important thing parents refer back to for support during labor and childbirth.

I will never forget an email I received from a woman who was the first of her class to give birth. She wrote to me and asked that I share her words with the rest of her still-pregnant classmates. What Natalie shared says a lot about what stuck with her from our classes together and what became relevant in labor. Here was the core of her email: "The Story of Inanna is NO F**KING JOKE. It is not a metaphor. It is REAL LIFE. Ladies, you will see her. You will become her. Bananas!"

I use the story of Inanna with the intention of helping parents prepare for the possibility that events in labor, birth, and new parenthood might not go as expected or planned, and as a powerful metaphor for the death/rebirth of the initiatory journey of birth. As a result, I take liberties and make variations from the original text.[3]

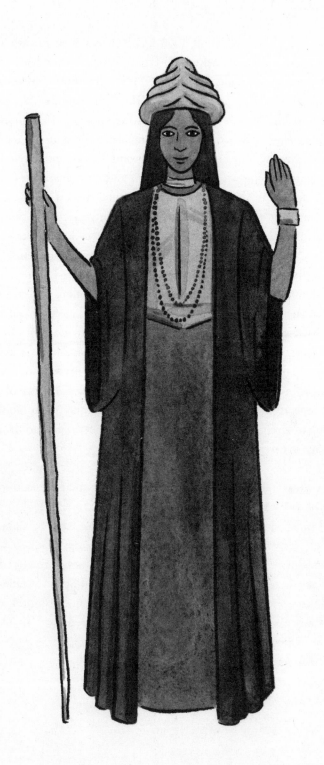

Inanna dates back to about 3000 BC, a time similar to that of the more familiar story of Gilgamesh.[4] The Sumerian people lived in the Fertile Crescent in Mesopotamia between the Tigris and Euphrates rivers, in what is present day Iraq and Kuwait. The Sumerians are often placed in history as "the creators of civilization as we know it." Their profound accomplishments included ancient written language and the establishment of the twenty-four-hour day, sixty-second minute, and sixty-minute hour.[5] Inanna was known to the Akkadians and Assyrians as the goddess Ishtar. I share all of this to give a bit of cultural context and respectful acknowledgment to the roots from whence Inanna comes, millennia before the myth became a fundamental part of my childbirth classes.

I like to share this story in two parts: the first maps the prenatal journey, and the second the postpartum experience. Before I share the first part of the story, I want to encourage you to follow along with the story in a personal way. To do so, you will need seven small pieces of paper and a pen (I use small sticky notes for the parents in my classes). On each piece of paper write one thing you imagine will be helpful to you in labor. Examples might be music, a tub or shower, touch or massage, movement, an epidural, your doula or partner . . . you get the idea. Write one of these helpful tools on each piece of paper and then number them randomly from one to seven and keep them nearby until they come into the story. Once you have written them, read on.

I want you to imagine we are sitting together around a fire with other parents-to-be. It's dark except for the light of the fire illuminating the faces of those gathered. In my classes, while I cannot have a campfire due to fire regulations, I do have a homemade "campfire" crafted of tissue paper "flames" and battery-operated candles. It might be helpful as you read this story to dim the lights and light a candle so that you too can mimic the ritual space that is created around a fire. Join me as we enter that otherworldly place of story now.

The Descent of Inanna, Part I

I'm going to tell you a story, an ancient story, a story about a queen. And this queen lived in a land far away, in a time long ago. Her name was Inanna. She was known as the Queen of Heaven and Earth. She was a strong and powerful woman, not all that different from you and me; you might even say she was the equivalent of a successful modern woman. She was organized, powerful, and in control of her well-ordered life.

One day, she hears a call, a call to visit the Underworld, to go to the place of the Great Below—the domain of the unconscious—to see what she has not yet seen, to experience what she has not yet experienced, to learn what she does not yet know, to head into the mystery.

"Inanna."

"Inaaanna!"

"Inaaannaaa!" The voice from the Underworld continues to call to her. She cannot ignore it.

Each of us hears calls in our own lives, the inner urgings toward a different adventure or a longing to know and experience something new. The Underworld represents this mysterious encounter with the unknown. It is neither inherently evil nor inherently good; rather it is something *other* that exists beyond duality and definition. Some say this indefinable and unknowable Underworld quality is a lot like birth and parenthood. Both reside in an unknowable land of great mystery.

The "call" to your Underworld journey might have manifested as a deep desire to have a child. Perhaps you had a desire to become a parent that started out as a little sound, just an inkling really, a voice that said, "I want to be a mother" or "I want to be a father." Or maybe the call came crashing into your life with an unexpected positive pregnancy test. However you were called to this journey, there is no going back now. Inanna, too, could not deny the pull toward the Great Below. The call had to be answered. She must venture into unknown lands, just as you will travel unfamiliar paths to and through birth.

Inanna begins to ready herself for the journey to the land of the unknown. She puts on her crown, fashioned from the horns of a great bull. The crown symbolizes her status and power as the Queen of Heaven and Earth. She places the crown upon her head, as she knows that whatever she faces, she will need the authority granted to her by that crown.

She puts her lapis necklace around her throat, adorning her center of speech. She adorns her body with the beauty of a double strand of beads, like those one would wear to a formal event. She puts on her breastplate, the one she wears to protect the most vital of all the organs—her heart. She armors herself to prevent being pierced or irreversibly wounded. Many of us also armor our hearts so that we don't feel things too deeply, thinking such shields will protect us from pain. She slips a gold circlet around her wrist. In the time of Inanna, gold was not something you picked up from a store on the corner. Gold was revered for its strength and flexibility, and was likely passed down, generation to generation, sort of the way birth stories are passed down. She covers her body with her royal cloak, protecting her from the elements and covering her body modestly. In the Upperworld, such clothing identifies her place among the civilized, cultured beings, marks her as socially acceptable, and sets her apart from the lowest of creatures and animals. She gathers her measuring rod and with it her ability to judge and discern good from bad. Tools of judgment often join us on journeys to unfamiliar places.

She is ready.

Inanna's faithful servant and friend, Ninshubur had helped Inanna get ready. Looking at Inanna, all dressed in her glorious regalia, Ninshubur becomes curious.

"Inanna, where are you going?"

"I am going to the Underworld to see what I have not yet seen, to learn what I do not yet know, to experience what I have not yet experienced."

Ninshubur becomes concerned. "Inanna, you can't go! Don't you know that no one returns from the Underworld unchanged?!"

Ninshubur is right; no one comes back from an experience of this magnitude unchanged. All of us have Ninshubur voices, within us or outside of us, that remind us to take care and do what needs to be done. These are the voices that remind us to turn off the iron or stove before we go out. In birth, these are the voices that may ask, "Are you sure? What if . . . ? Have you thought about . . . ?"

Inanna, in her wisdom, gives Ninshubur a task.

"Ninshubur, faithful friend, will you watch for my return and if after three days I have not returned, put on your sackcloth of grief, bang the drums, gather my community, and tell them what has happened to me? Then go to the elders and ask them to help bring me back. Will you do this for me?"

"Yes, my Queen," Ninshubur replies.

In giving Ninshubur this task, Inanna has turned her friend's concern into useful support; turned her worry into something that will help them both. Often those around us who express concern need a task to focus on instead of dwelling on their worry. When they feel they can be helpful or useful they are able to relax more around their own anxiety. In your life this might be giving a concerned in-law the job of making and freezing meals for the time after birth or asking them to pray for you while you are in labor. Tasks can be simple or more complex, practical or spiritual.

And in giving Ninshubur this task, Inanna has also done something that every adventurer must do; she has planned for her return. In so doing, she has freed herself for the journey ahead.

Inanna begins her journey, setting out toward the Underworld. But she comes to a gate blocking her way. This is strange and unexpected to Inanna, as she has encountered few obstacles before. She knocks on the gate.

From the other side of the gate comes a voice. The gatekeeper, Neti, asks, "Who are you and why have you come?"

"I am Inanna, Queen of Heaven and Earth. Let me in. I have come to learn what I do not yet know, to experience what I have not yet experienced, to see what I have not seen."

"Stay here. I will talk with my queen."

Neti zips down through the labyrinth of the Underworld to where his queen, Ereshkigal, is sitting on her throne. He says to her, "My queen, my queen, you'll never guess who's at the gate. Inanna, Queen of Heaven and Earth."

When Ereshkigal hears this, she slaps her thigh and bites her lip. She takes the matter into her heart and thinks about it.

It is important to know that Ereshkigal and Inanna are sisters. You could say they are two sides of the same coin. Inanna is the social self, the part of us we share more publicly, while Ereshkigal is our unexpressed side, that part of us we share with no one, or almost no one. Inanna lives boldly in the Upperworld for all to see. Ereshkigal lives in the hidden darkness of the Underworld. These two sisters made an agreement long ago that Inanna would live in the Upperworld while

Ereshkigal would live in the Underworld, just as we make decisions about what part of ourselves we let others know.

Ereshkigal speaks. "Neti, here is what you are to do. Bolt the seven gates. At each gate take something of value from her. Let the high queen enter, humbled."

"Yes, my queen." And with that, Neti bolts the gates and zips back up to the first gate where Inanna is waiting . . . not too patiently.

Neti opens the first gate and snatches from Inanna her crown.

"What is this?!" Inanna cries.

"Quiet, Inanna. The ways of the Underworld are tried, true, and ancient. Carry on."

Reader: Take your note numbered one and toss it away. Neti just took this from you, and, like Inanna, you will continue forward without it. You may not like it and may resist it, fight it, or just brush it off. Pause and ask yourself, "How will I keep going without this thing I thought I needed?"

Inanna has to question who she is without her crown, without her ability to use her royal powers and status to influence events, just as you have to question who you are, as you make this descent into the unknown. In the Underworld, all travelers are equal.

Inanna isn't too worried about her crown. She keeps going toward the Underworld. As she continues, she begins to think about where she might find or make another crown. We do this too; we negotiate with ourselves, we try to recreate that which has been taken from us, fight against its removal, or try to figure out ways to keep going without it.

Inanna continues and comes to more gates, and at each gate Neti takes something of value from her: her lapis necklace, double strand of beads, and gold circlet. Slowly and steadily, she is stripped of more of her special adornments.

Reader: Take number two, three, and four of your notes and toss them away. Neti just took these from you, and, like Inanna, you will have to continue without them. Notice what comes up for you as these items are stripped away. What do you have to do to keep going even without that which you thought you needed?

Who is Inanna without her necklace that hangs around her throat, giving her voice? Who are you if you do not have access to the usual Upperworld strength of your voice? Who is Inanna without her beads and jewelry? Down here, in the Underworld, the experience is rarely dressed up and fancy. Even when births are captured in stunning pictures by talented photographers, birth seldom *feels* beautiful in the moment. It is a personal experience that does not need to be adorned for anyone else. Inanna's Underworld experience is hers, just as your birth journey will be yours.

Even without the familiar adornments of the Upperworld, Inanna must continue, just like you will have to do. She isn't feeling as bold or righteous as she was when she began. She hadn't counted on the gates. The path is difficult. The further she descends, the darker it gets. Before long, she comes to another gate and reluctantly knocks.

Neti asks, "Who are you?"

Inanna is less bold this time and answers, "I am . . . Inanna? I can hardly remember now what I have come for."

Neti opens the door taking from Inanna her breastplate.

"Wait, what?"

"Ahhh, Inanna, the ways of the Underworld contain ancient wisdom. Carry on."

Reader: Take number five of your notes and toss it away. Neti just took this from you, and, like Inanna, you don't have to like it, and you might even fight it or argue with yourself or others about it. Pay attention to what you need to do to keep going without whatever was on your piece of paper.

Without her breastplate, Inanna's heart is exposed. She can now feel and be hurt. She is capable of experiencing depths of feeling she has never before known. She is no longer participating as if watching, but rather an active, emotional part of the journey itself.

But the journey is hard, harder than she expected. The walls of the labyrinth are closing in. Roots of the trees above are poking into the path, and Inanna's cloak is catching on them while she travels deeper and deeper within.

She has to get down on all fours to continue forward. It's getting sticky and gooey as things drip down from the walls and ceiling. She has to almost close her eyes to continue. It is slower now too—there is no rushing. She takes her time, one hand, one foot in front of the other, step by step. At one point, Inanna stops. She doesn't think she can go on. She looks back up the way she's come, wondering if she can go back. But all the gates have closed behind her. The only way is forward. It feels like too much.

She stops. She sits. She waits.

It doesn't matter how long she sits. She can wait for as long as it takes. At some point she knocks on the next gate. She might gather her determination from deep within and start walking to the next gate, or without knowing it, she's next to the gate and perhaps from exhaustion leans into it unintentionally knocking on it. Regardless of what inspires her to keep going, Neti is there, ready for her.

"Who are you, and why have you come to the land from which no one returns unmarked or unchanged?"

"I am Inanna. Just Inanna."

"Ah, you are getting closer."

Neti opens the gate and takes from Inanna her royal cloak, baring her whole body.

Reader: Take number six of your notes and toss it away. Neti just took this from you, and, like Inanna, you will have to find a way to continue without it. How will you do that?

Without much conviction, Inanna says, "Oh, please. Not that."

Neti responds, "Carry on, Inanna."

Inanna does. She is surprised to find that it is actually a bit easier without her cloak. No longer is it catching and snagging on the roots and rocks along the path. She hardly cares that her body is bare, as she has become so engrossed in the rhythmic motion of hand, knee, hand, knee, hand, knee. It is almost as if thinking has become too great an effort. She is moving forward, and that is all.

She doesn't know how many gates are left or how many she's already passed through. Time and quantifiable things like numbers of gates have no meaning down here. She has entered another realm. The Underworld, like labor, is a different land, a different consciousness, almost an altered reality by means of it being *too real*. Inanna is no longer the woman she knew herself to be before she started this journey. The social identity she wore in the Upperworld ceases to be. She has become the process itself. She is just *this*.

Coming to the last gate, Neti asks, "Who are you?"

Inanna answers, "I am this."

Neti takes from her the measuring rod. There is nothing to measure down here anyway. The judges are different in the Underworld. The Upperworld tools for judgment have no use down here. Societal rules for acceptable behavior have no bearing in this land below and in the land of birth as well.

Reader: Look at number seven of your notes and ask if you really need it. What if Neti let you choose whether or not to toss it away? How would that make it different to you? Decide if you will keep this or toss it along with the others. Regardless of what you decide, ask yourself who you are without it.

Inanna enters through the final gate naked, bare, and humbled. She enters into the throne room of her sister, the Queen of the Underworld. Ereshkigal sits upon her throne and looks on Inanna with the Eye of Death. In that moment Inanna dies.

Inanna dies, but you could say this is what it is like when you look into the eyes of your newborn child for the first time. Some part of you is gone forever. You can never go back to a time before that specific gaze altered you, to a time before those eyes pierced your heart. Something in you is changed with that single glance. It is difficult to express the profound change that comes over you when you see or hold your baby for the first time. Some say it feels like a kind of death, a death of who you were before. It is as if we mark our lives in two parts—the time before we became a parent and the time after—two different selves separated by this one profound moment.

But Ereshkigal doesn't care about all this. She motions to her guards and says, "Hang her on the hook." The guards pick up the corpse of Inanna and hang it on a hook.

This is where we are going to leave Inanna for now. We will return to her a little later as this is not the end of her story.

•

It is common in my classes for parents to be teary or outright crying by the time we get to the end of this segment of the story. They express frustration and excitement that I've left them, like Inanna, hanging on the hook until later. Emotions are a good thing, here and in labor.

Invite the story to work on you. But don't try to "figure it out" or try to have it make sense in your rational mind. Remember that stories don't work like that. Instead of doing anything to it or about it, let yourself marinate in the images and story elements. Notice where you entered the story. In other words, notice where you were captivated, repulsed, or curious. These might be important story points to explore further.

Parents often tell me how after hearing this story, they talked with their partner the whole way home from class. Or they share how they found thoughts of Inanna popping up throughout their week. Some people even share how the story enters their dreams at night. Story works in different ways and on various planes of consciousness. Roll with it and be curious! As a parent, you'll need to be well versed at navigating fantasy and story because the imaginal realm is where children live for the first several years of their lives.

Elements from the story may show up in your mind over the course of the next week or so. You might never think of it again. Or it might show up for you in labor like a ladder upon which to hang some of your experiences and help give them context. Sometimes it is only after you have faced a few of your own "gates" that you may truly feel the impact of the story on your life. With story, there is nothing you need to do to "get it."

I remember a mom who did a *lot* in preparation for her first birth, including taking my classes. She wanted to create exactly the birth she desired and believed that lots of preparation would make that happen. As it turned out, she had an experience in labor that closely resembled her hopes for it. She believed she had created her experience by doing the "right" things she had learned prenatally (and maybe she had, who can know). However, when she faced unexpected challenges with breastfeeding soon after birth, it was not the skills learned in preparation, not the breathing techniques or the information about labor, or even what she had learned about breastfeeding that helped her through this challenge. It was the story of Inanna. Remembering this story helped her make sense of the struggle she was facing. She hit gates in postpartum, and the story of Inanna's descent came to mind and guided her through. She kept asking herself, "How do I keep going even without this that I thought I needed?"

Let's reflect a bit further on the story. What happened when Inanna's cloak was taken from her? Did you notice how without it she was able to move more easily even though she was certain she would need that item of clothing on her journey? Sometimes grasping tightly to what we were sure we would need is what keeps us catching on the roots of the Underworld. Sometimes, letting go of our expectations is what allows us to move more freely, as was the case with Inanna and her cloak.

This can happen in labor too. I witnessed a woman who was certain she would not use an epidural. She had decided this without wavering. She struggled and fought with her own desire to birth naturally for many hours. Deep in labor her progress stalled. At one point, she felt herself surrender her ideas about "doing it right" and asked for an epidural. Something magical happened after that. She was able to relax around the contractions, and her labor kicked back into gear. It was as if the energy spent *resisting* the contractions and *resisting* the epidural was keeping her cervix closed. Once she opened her mind to another way, her body followed suit. Sometimes, when we let go of the metaphoric cloak, we discover it's actually been making our experience more difficult.

What was your experience with letting go of your personal support items, the ones you wrote on the small pieces of paper? Were there any that didn't make sense or confused you? Okay, maybe it made sense when music was taken from you, but what about your doula or partner? Surely, *they* would always be there, and it wouldn't be possible for the gatekeeper of birth to strip you of them. But might it be possible that someone you expect to be a comfort and support to you turns out not to be the help you imagined? Is it possible that even those people physically present aren't the support you expected? Or, maybe you put "love" or "God" on your piece of paper and they got taken. How could that be? Here's the thing: even our faith and love can be tested in labor and birth. That doesn't mean they aren't actually there for you, but your ability to access connection with them can be challenged.

The bigger question then becomes, how do you keep going even if aspects you most expected to be supportive aren't? Stretch yourself to explore what it would take for you to keep going even if those things you put on your scraps of paper aren't helpful. Rather than spending time clutching them tightly, expand your ability to keep going regardless of what happens. If letting go of an item of support triggered an emotional reaction in you, spend some time with that, exploring ways to rally whatever is needed to resiliently proceed forward.

Inanna is prepared. She is ready. She has all that she knows she will need. And still she is surprised. Still she meets unexpected challenges. Still she must let go of expectations and ideas of who she is. Most important, however, Inanna must keep going even after the items she was sure she needed have been taken from her. You will need to keep going too, even if what you think will be helpful isn't, or events prevent you from even being able to use them. Each aspect of this story is ripe for exploration.

Identity Death No One Talks About

Fear of actual death in childbirth makes exploring any type of death tricky at best. But for birth to fulfill its potential as an initiation into a new identity, many precious aspects of our previous identity must die in the process. Becoming a parent is perhaps the most deeply significant rite of passage most human beings will go through. We must die to one phase of our lives and the roles associated with that period and enter a new stage with a new identity. Childbirth, particularly with first births, involves a very clear ending of one chapter and the beginning of another.

The identity change involves awakening to secrets unique to parents and being invited into the cliquish club of parenthood. New parents are invited into the club of parents only *after* giving birth. Prior to birth, pregnancy places parents in the liminal space between not yet a parent and full parenthood. Similarly, adoptive parents are invited in, but again, only after their baby is in arms and not during the period of "almost" parenthood. It is the process of undergoing the ordeals of initiation and experiencing the psychic death that are required. Pregnancy often makes people unsure of where they fit in. Other parents look at them with knowing looks as if to say, "Oh, honey, I know what you're about to face," but don't really see them as one of them, at least not yet.

The change in identity is so encompassing that the individual steps into a new role and receives a new name; they become "parent," "mother," "father," or take on some other new name. But the transformation is more than simply the taking on of a new name; it is embracing a new identity, one that requires communications to be signed with "Love, Mom" and phone calls to begin with "Hi Sweetie, it's Dad." For at least the first ten years of my motherhood journey and perhaps longer, it was considerably more common to hear myself addressed as Mom than as Britta. While my *role* with my children was as their mother, my *name* had changed. To them, I am known and referred to not as Britta but as Mom. Giving a new name to the initiate immediately following rites of initiation is common. I can't think of another time in a modern person's life when they will so completely embrace a new identity, including being renamed. Part of the regeneration process is the death of a familiar identity and the rebirth of a new self.

REBIRTH

Fear and resistance of the death aspect of the regeneration cycle has created a culture where death is denied but still occurring. But when we deny it and fail to give it an appropriate place within cyclical existence, we also cut ourselves off from the other half of the regenerative cycle, that of rebirth. That is what the second part of Inanna's story is all about.

The Descent of Inanna, Part II

Let us remember that Ninshubur is waiting in the Upperworld for Inanna's return. After three days, the queen has not returned. Ninshubur puts on her sackcloth of grief, bangs her drum, and gets the community engaged to help bring Inanna back. Then, she goes to the elders for help.

The first two elders she meets won't help. One is too busy to help, and the other disagrees with Inanna's choice to go to the Underworld to begin with and now believes she should live with the consequences. These sorts of responses sometimes happen. People can have too much going on in their own lives or judgment might cloud their ability to help you.

Undeterred, Ninshubur continues on to the next elder. To this one she says, "Please help us. Your daughter Inanna has gone to the Underworld and has not returned. You must help her."

The elder responds, "Sit down my child and tell me what has happened."

While Ninshubur tells him of Inanna's troubles, the elder cleans the dirt from under his fingernails.

Ninshubur asks, "How can you do that at a time like this?"

"Ah," said the elder, "don't assume that what is mundane lacks significance. It is often the simplest of gestures that make the greatest difference." And from the dirt under his nails he creates two wingless creatures: the kurgarra and the galatur. He gives them the food and water of life.

Then he says, "Go to the Underworld. There, you will find the Queen of the Underworld suffering. Comfort her. She will offer you gifts in thanks. Accept only the corpse of Inanna."

The kurgarra and the galatur zip down through the labyrinth of the Underworld totally undetected by Neti. And just as the elder had told them, they are gifted the corpse of Inanna by the Underworld queen.

But let's remember, the corpse of Inanna has been hanging on the hook for three days and three nights. She doesn't look too good! Her corpse has been left to rot. She lacks all muscle tone. She's flabby and lifeless. But external looks can be deceiving, because the true transformation is occurring inside and may not be visible to the world outside. Inside, Inanna has been transfiguring, much as a caterpillar turns into a butterfly. Parts of her are dissolving and becoming goo. This dissolution of her old self is necessary before she can be reformed as the person she needs to become. The work of becoming a parent transfigures us. The process is rarely visible from the outside, and when it is, it isn't pretty.

The kurgarra and the galatur feed Inanna the food of life. This is symbolic of practical sustenance like having someone to do the mountains of laundry, bring food, and help with tending to the baby's needs. They sprinkle her with the water of life, which you could say, is like bathing her in emotional support. These are the things that tend to her soul, like someone to listen to her tell her story or rub her feet or hold the baby so she can rest and heal.

Fed the food and the water of life, Inanna jumps back to life and heads for the door. She's ready to go! But there, the guards of the Underworld stop her. No one is allowed to leave unmarked or unchanged. She is not allowed to depart without leaving something or someone in her place. In the original myth, Inanna takes a long time to decide who shall go in her place, but in the end, she selects her husband. Some couples feel like they swap places in the Underworld!

Every parent on their return leaves something of value in the Underworld while they make their journey out. This might be a course of study, a career, or something as simple as a clean car (I'm still wondering when I will get that back!). Something must be left behind, at least temporarily. Sometimes you know ahead of time exactly what that will be, and sometimes you're surprised.

As Inanna begins her ascent, she must stop at each gate and take inventory of what she left there. She must ask herself if what was stripped away is of value to her now. She may see the breastplate that she discarded on her descent and decide that armoring her heart is no longer the way she wishes to live. Step by step Inanna climbs higher, getting ever-closer to the land above. This journey can take a short time or a long time. It can start and stop many times. It has twists and turns, openings and closings. But, after a time she does make it out.

Inanna is changed. She has gathered new knowing and come out transfigured. Just as you will make your descent to find what you do not yet know and be touched in ways you have not yet felt, you will also ascend, making your way out of the Underworld step by step, becoming more of who you are meant to be every moment. By the time you ascend to the Upperworld again, you will be different. You will be changed. Others may or may not even notice. Much of who you have known yourself to be can be found again on the journey up. Some of it has been forever altered. Your task is to walk your unique path down, die to your former identity, receive the help of the allies, and make your ascent to discover who you are after you have been transformed by birth.

You Do Not
Have to
Be Perfect

In this Apollonian culture where predictability and order are prized, the wildness of the birthing body seems to defy control and perfection. If perfection means measuring up to an ideal based on established norms made within a mechanistic society, the body is a faulty machine with parts that break, programing that goes haywire, and formulas that confound the scientific method that says one plus two should always equal three, every time. Science relies on the ability to reproduce results on different days, by different people, in different situations. In a culture where the scientific method is key to our understanding and where, in the age of computers, formulas entered exactly the same way time and again produce the same results, the variability and unpredictability of childbearing and parenting can be befuddling. Instead of questioning whether the ability to reproduce results is a flawed system for dealing with something as unpredictable and unique as a personal body, our cultural adoration of certainty keeps medical providers, birth professionals, and parents looking for ever-better formulas to impose on birthing people in order to create the illusion of reliable results.

Be wary of the belief that your choices, education, and strategies *create certainty*. These things can help *influence* events, but cannot guarantee specific outcomes or provide certainty, no matter how badly you desire it. Some of the most traumatized parents I've known are those planning and expecting an out-of-hospital birth but then have to transfer to a hospital and have a cesarean instead. The radical difference between expectation and experience is so vast, it rocks emotional bedrock. That doesn't mean that you shouldn't continue with your personal intentions and desires for birth. What it does mean is that just because you're planning a particular type of birth does not guarantee that that's the type of birth you'll have; nor does it eliminate the possibility of having to navigate a birth totally different from what you desire.

THE QUEST FOR PERFECTION

Parenthood tests the drive for perfection in profound ways. Children live outside of your body and yet feel like a part of you. Other people, outside events, and your own reactions and behavior collectively create the reality of any situation. In the best case, you only have control over your behavior, but even that is questionable.

When I came across the Michael Sandel passage I shared in chapter 3, it perfectly expressed this relationship between parenthood and perfection, particularly the phrase "openness to the unbidden," which stopped me in my tracks. Yes! That's the profound lesson of parenthood. Parenthood teaches us to be open to that which we do not ask for or desire. I would argue that it is precisely because of its ability to teach us to be open to the unbidden that parenthood has been called one of the greatest spiritual practices. It is through facing imperfection and the illusion of control that we are reminded we are not God, we are merely human.

Sandel also says, "In a social world that prizes mastery and control, parenthood is a school for humility. That we care deeply about our children, and yet cannot choose the kind we want, teaches us to be open to the unbidden. Such openness is a disposition worth affirming, not only within families but in the wider world as well. It invites us to abide the unexpected, to live with dissonance, to rein in the impulse to control."[1]

If it is parenthood that teaches us to be open, then birth is the beginning of that education. Birth, and our inability to design it to our specifications, begins the important humbling process of surrender. We do not need yet another method for control but rather a new paradigm that embraces the power of surrender, resilience, and growth. There is power in letting go: "What is required on our part is nothing less than active attention, a willing renunciation of willing."[2]

Willing renunciation of willing is what Zoe and Jamie had to practice in their birth. They knew early on in their pregnancy that they wanted to work with a midwife and have a home or birth-center birth. As a birth professional herself, Zoe knew which midwife to hire to support the "best birth." When that midwife didn't seem to give them the attention they wanted, they hired a different midwife. That midwife didn't work out for them either. They interviewed others, visited birth centers, and kept looking. By the time they hired a well-known obstetrician who works at a major Los Angeles hospital, they had gone through several different providers hunting for the right one for them. Zoe surprised herself in deciding on a hospital birth, learning that what she thought was best as a birth professional conflicted with the gravitational pull she felt as a pregnant woman. It took her as long as it did to find the provider that felt best to her in large part because what she really wanted was so different from what she thought she *should* want. Letting go came in the form of letting go of expectations about what "doing it right" looked like.

For Zoe, and for many parents, the rite of passage of parenthood included letting go of external measurements or her own preconceived ideas and tuning in deeply to her own inner truth in the moment. Gold stars given for doing well on someone else's scale have no value. You must find your own way, your personal truth, now and in parenthood.

EXCEPTIONALISM

Exceptionalism is a shadow aspect of perfectionism that runs through Western culture (particularly upper-middle-class white culture). This is the belief that our way is the best. This thread is woven, like independence, throughout the history of the West, especially in the United States. Exceptionalism is part of what fueled colonialism—the belief that "I have the answers and it is my duty to share them with those who don't know."

This ideal is visible in the desire to export modern birth technologies abroad without concern for what cultural practices might be lost upon their implementation. It is also visible in the profound denial that something might be wrong in our birth culture and that parents, especially those of color, are still dying in childbirth at alarming rates. If this culture were not built on exceptionalism, there would be more overt curiosity about how others do things, about what works elsewhere; there would be less racism, sexism, and classism, and humility would be present.

In ancient Greece, this idea was called "hubris" and referred to a declaration of being better than the gods. Greek mythology is full of famous stories of hubris and its consequences. One particular one comes to mind from Ovid's *Metamorphoses*.[3] The story involves the very talented weaver Arachne who boasted that she was a better weaver than Athena, the goddess of crafts, including weaving. Arachne's claim infuriated Athena, as all claims of hubris did, and the goddess punished Arachne by turning her into a spider.

Hubris is poisonous. We don't need any God-given punishment to feel its toxicity. Exceptionalism is the hubristic idea that we know best, universally, for all, like Arachne claimed about weaving. Exceptionalism is rampant in parenting culture today. All you have to do is join a social media group targeting parents and read the comments. Almost everyone has "the answer." The hubris is on full display, and its toxicity permeates outward into parenting realms like an airborne poison. Sadly, and perhaps paradoxically, hubris almost always keeps us stuck in the insecurity or inadequacy that it's trying to pull us out of.

The two ideals, perfectionism and exceptionalism, fuel nearly all the conflict in the mommy wars. What is lacking is true humility.

GROUNDED HUMILITY

Humility is one of the great lessons of parenthood. Grounded humility is the antidote to perfectionism and exceptionalism. Understanding birth as a rite of passage gives context for the struggles, unraveling, and challenges that confront our ideals of perfectionism and exceptionalism. Each journey is unique and personal. There are no universal truths.

Becoming uniquely yourself is important, but aim for genuine, not perfect. Hopefully, as long as we are alive, we are growing. True personal growth is not an outward journey. Striving for perfection and engaging in personal growth are two separate things that should not be conflated. When determination is healthy it aims for growth and improvement over time, not some pinnacle of achievement where we plant our flag and announce our arrival at the top! There is no top. It is not our job to climb, or even aspire to climb, the Mount Everest of birth or life. Life and the journey into parenthood are more like a mountain *range* with many peaks and valleys rather than a single destination. As soon as we make it to the top of one challenge, there is another one waiting for us.

Focusing on the Future

Often, we focus on what we *don't* want and how to avoid it. This is sort of like driving a car while looking in the rearview mirror. While the rearview mirror is helpful and an important tool in driving, unless we wish to go backward, it's not where we want our focus to be while moving *forward*. Instead, we have to locate how we wish to be in the future and move in the direction of our desired destination.

 Try This

Crafting Your Personal Question

The practice of crafting and using a personal question can be very powerful for those on the threshold of birth or life transition or those looking for transformation. I originally learned this practice from Pam England, but its origins are in Zen practice.[4] The idea with this practice is to engage with the question, to explore what can't be understood intellectually and grow from the act of asking it. Asking your question should guide you *inward* to seek the answer not from information, but from moving, acting, and *living* into your life as you want it to be right now, rather than at some distant time.

Try writing a "How am I . . ." question rather than a "Can I . . ." question. "Can I . . ." questions beg for a yes or no answer rather than personal exploration. Write your question in the present tense. For example, one person's question might look like this: "How am I embracing the unexpected in this moment?" Another might be, "How am I holding myself tenderly in this moment?" Or, "How am I being the person I wish to be right now?"

There is no formula, but this structure can help some who struggle to craft their desired inward shift into a question. You want your question to send you seeking *how* you are already moving in the direction you wish to grow.

Once you have crafted your question, begin using it. Try writing your question on sticky notes and placing them in areas where you will see them as you go about your day. For me, that includes my bathroom mirror, the refrigerator, and the dashboard of my car.

Ask yourself your personal question and notice where in your life *you are already doing what you wish to create*. The idea with this practice is to water what you want to grow. Noticing what's already working helps to strengthen that muscle, encouraging it to grow further. Use your question to focus your attention out the front windshield rather than driving the vehicle of your life by looking in the rearview mirror. Focus forward in the direction of what's working, where you wish to go, and the change you want to see in your life.

Asking yourself a well-crafted personal question guides you toward the future you desire, growing skills all along the way.

SURRENDER AND LETTING GO

Navigating an ordeal of initiation often requires more than modern parents are prepared to give. For some, enduring the intensity of labor with strength and determination is enough. These parents "power through," challenged by pain, the need for endurance, and a deep-down gritty force of will. In natural birth circles, these are the images most often shared of what it takes to get through the potency of labor.

However, often, the price extracted at the crossroads of birth comes as deep surrender, having to let go of the image of a "perfect birth" (whatever that is for each individual), and a death of some part of who the birthing individual thought they were. Everyone who experiences an initiatory journey, one that readies them for rebirth, must make a payment or offer a sacrifice to pass through to the other side. In Greek mythology, souls must cross from the land of the living to the Underworld or Hades, by crossing the River Styx. To get across they had to make a payment to the ferryman, Charon. Everyone makes some sort of payment to get across the threshold of birth. There is a sacrifice required. The word *sacrifice* actually means "to make sacred."

Initiation through childbirth is not limited to natural birth. There are various possible thresholds to cross during initiatory passages. A desired natural birth that instead requires the involvement of technology and medical support does not automatically default the entire process to the category of failed passage . . . far from it!

In practice, initiatory ordeals take many forms. For many, it is facing the intensity of labor, but it can also be asking for medical support, including pain medicine, that acts as the ordeal for others. Asking for help can sometimes be as difficult as or even more difficult than "toughing it out." Very often, surrender of an idealized image shapes the initiatory ordeal. Birth does not always (or even often) fit some idealized image of initiation. Initiation by definition is not always magical, beautiful, or ideal. The initiatory ordeal can take many different paths. Katrina's birth is a good example.

Katrina arrived in my childbirth classes with flowing hair and tattooed arms. She was already highly prepared for the home birth she was planning. Unlike some mothers I have worked with, Katrina was realistic about what giving birth without pain medicine would ask of her. She was heading into the process with intentionality, personal fortitude, and a deep willingness to surrender to the oceanic waves of labor. She and her husband, Jesse, had educated themselves and learned much about the birth process, equipping themselves with information and goals. However, their ordeal was different from what they thought it would be.

This naturally minded couple was hit late in pregnancy with the knowledge that there was an issue: an ultrasound detected placenta previa, a condition where the placenta covers, or partially covers, the opening of the cervix. Placenta previa is one of the few rarely contested reasons to birth via a planned cesarean. Katrina and Jesse were devastated. They were ready and excited for the rite of passage through labor and birth. But they had never given a thought to birthing surgically. The ordeal they confronted involved deep emotional stress provoked by having to let go of their idealized image of a home birth.

Katrina and Jesse were taking my classes and preparing for birth as an initiatory process when they got this news. Connecting with birth as a rite of passage helped them to frame their experience in a meaningful way. Katrina looked at her birth through *The Descent of Inanna*, seeing the loss of a home birth as one of the items stripped from her by the gatekeeper on her unique journey. Rather than asking, "Why did this happen?" Katrina and her husband asked, "How can we keep going and make our birth the very best it can be?" Like Inanna, they continued toward the Underworld even after an unexpected medical condition stripped them of their imagined birth before labor even started. And they did not have to be happy about what they had lost. In fact, they mourned the loss of their desired birth, they cried, and they got angry, all while simultaneously knowing that they could move forward with the birth they were given in the best way possible. Ultimately, they were thrilled at the arrival of their son, open to the way he needed to be born, and sad at the loss of their wished-for birth. They were able to hold multiple truths at *the same time*.

Childbirth tests the notion that perfection not only exists but also is attainable through correct action. Birth reminds us that control is illusory. Katrina and Jesse did everything they thought was "right" and still gave birth surgically. Labor and birth mess with our basic understanding of how things work and what we believe to be true. It is in part due to this disruption of familiar elements that consciousness in birth shifts from the mundane to the sacred.

The coin placed in Charon's hand to cross the initiatory threshold regularly involves a strength born from deepest vulnerability rather than might. Perfectionism is an attempt to protect us from feeling the vulnerability that is inherent in a process as transformative as giving birth. It is in these moments of surrender that control loses its grip. It is no accident that the watery initiation of childbirth most often requires a dropping down into the depths of darkness, into chaos, where order and control have no power. It is there where birthing people are tested through an unknowable initiation that includes a metamorphosis of the self.

UNWELCOME SURPRISES IN LABOR AND BIRTH

Transformative rites of passage can, and often do, include unwelcome surprises and ordeals that profoundly challenge you. Perfection is an illusion. Mystery is inherent in birth. You can't know ahead of time exactly what you will face. What you can know is that something along the path to parenthood, be it in pregnancy, birth, or postpartum, will test you. Katrina and Jesse's test came as an unexpected cesarean as I shared before, others are challenged in breastfeeding, while still others face the need to ask for help during labor, be it for pain or to help kick-start a stalled labor. It isn't for you to figure out how you will be tested but to develop the resilience to face whatever comes. Everything addressed thus far in this book is designed to help you do exactly that.

Willingness to learn about cesareans and epidurals helps parents mature. It takes courage to face what you wish to avoid.

Epidurals

We already discussed a little bit about epidurals during the section on pain in chapter 6, but there are a few additional pieces to explore.

An epidural is a local anesthetic that is inserted in the epidural space near the spinal column (see figure on the next page). A parent who has hoped to birth without this pain medication might be disappointed if they find they actually *want* it during labor. This is a place where the illusion of perfection can be tough to let go of. For some

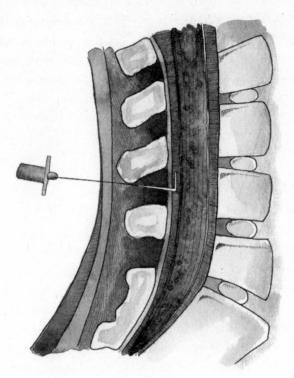

parents it is the act of *asking for help* that is the true lesson of their rite of passage into parenthood.

Parents committed to an unmedicated birth prior to labor, often want to know that they have given all they have before receiving pharmaceutical help. What can you do to help alleviate some of the doubt later about whether or not you did all you could without an epidural?

A few things can be helpful in this regard. First, laboring where epidurals aren't available makes getting one difficult! Out-of-hospital births put the possibility of an epidural farther out of reach, which in turn tends to help motivation to navigate labor without one. This means that if a parent needs an epidural, they know they *really* need it because they have to change many other factors in order to receive one. My sister, Alissa, lives in the backwoods of Northern California, and the drive to the birth center was one of the worst parts of her labor. She hated the car ride! At one point while laboring at the birthing center, she looked at me and said, "I want an epidural." I responded that we could absolutely get her one, we'd just have to get in the car and head to the hospital. She glowered at me and returned to labor. There was no way she wanted to get back in the car!

It can be trickier when epidurals are available on demand. Some couples come up with a code word that when used communicates, "I really mean it; I want an epidural." This allows the birthing parent to ask for one, like my sister did, without everyone jumping to make it happen when the birthing parent just wanted to be able to say, "I want an epidural!"

It can be really hard for partners, who may have heard for months "no epidural" to then know how to respond in labor if their partner asks for one. That can feel like a "damned if I do and damned if I don't" conundrum! What I recommend is what I learned from my teacher and have recommended to parents for nearly two decades: Listen to the request as a call for help. This sort of request, especially when counter to what has been hoped for, is a communication that labor is big; bigger than they can do alone, and they *need more help*.

Partners: turn toward this request with deep respect and renewed focus. Commit to working with your beloved for a set amount of time—thirty minutes, the next hour, five contractions—whatever feels right in the moment, but long enough that things might actually shift in that time and short enough that the birthing parent can imagine continuing that long. During that time, dedicate yourself completely to every moment, every contraction, every breath right by their side. Stay with them in body, heart, and attention. Give them more help. If after the agreed upon amount of time, the birthing parent still wants the epidural, help them get it. Frequently, the moment of asking for an epidural is the place of great doubt where the birthing parent doesn't know how to keep going without it. The focus and dedication of their partner or doula can often help get over that hump. If not, the parents can know they gave it everything they could *before* getting an epidural. This can help reduce "what ifs" after the fact.

If an epidural becomes a part of your birth experience, stay connected to your baby, to your birth journey, to yourself, to your partner, to the sacredness of the experience. Birth with an epidural can be a totally amazing and life-changing experience. What tends to happen after an epidural has been placed is that the energy of the room changes. Everyone's focus dissipates while they take care of themselves, since the epidural reduces the need for focused attention on the birthing parent and the task of labor. Instead of scattering the focus, stay connected to the process of labor continuing whether you feel it or not. Wrap up and rest or take a nap. Snuggle, hold hands, or kiss your partner. Have your partner or birth companion give you a foot rub. The intimate bubble of labor does not have to pop just because an epidural has been utilized. Remember that what really matters is how you are being with yourself and the experience and not what boxes you can check about what you did and didn't do in labor.

Cesarean Birth

About a third of all babies in the United States are born surgically. In some states, that number is lower, while for others it is higher. Rates also vary by provider and hospital. The World Health Organization, or WHO, states that the ideal rate for cesarean births is between 10 and 15 percent.[5]

There is a gap between this recommended rate and the cesarean rates around the world. The United States and Australian rates of cesarean are about 32 to 33 percent, Canada is about 26 percent, while in Egypt and Brazil over half of all babies are born surgically, and it is suspected that in private hospitals in South Africa the cesarean rate could be as high as 90 percent.[6] These numbers far surpass the upper end of the recommendation by WHO. Clearly, there is something going on here.

It's important to remember that cesareans can save lives. According to WHO, "studies show that when caesarean section rates rise toward 10 percent across a population, the number of maternal and newborn deaths decreases. When the rate goes above 10 percent, there is no evidence that mortality rates improve."[7] Let's break this down into plain speak. What these numbers mean is that 10 to 15 percent of births would end in death for either the parent or the baby if not for this life-saving surgery. Before this was an option and where it is still unavailable, babies and/or parents die when they could have been saved by a surgical birth. In the culture of idealized birth, these hard truths are often forgotten or at least ignored. It's important to include in the conversation the percentage of births for which this method of delivery saves lives.

Also missing from most conversations about cesareans is the word *birth*. Whether or not desired by the parents, about a third of babies in the United States are born this way. It is their birth. As such, I believe it important to include the word birth in the conversation.

When we use the term *C-section*, images of cutting, drapes, doctors, and blood tend to fill our mind. C-section sounds like something that is done to someone rather than a choice decided and agreed upon by the parent as the right next step. Returning the word *birth* helps shift the focus back to the one giving birth and the one being born. There are a few ways to incorporate birth into the name of this type of delivery. I most often use "surgical birth" or "cesarean birth" or "birth by cesarean." Others like to call it a "belly birth." Explore for yourself what feels right to you. Practice using this term when talking or asking questions about this type of birth with others.

Even though many conversations about cesareans are coupled with the word *emergency*, not all necessary, unexpected, and in-labor cesareans are true emergencies. To my mind, there are emergency cesarean births and necessary cesarean births, but the two are not always one and the same. The word *emergency* implies an urgent need for immediate action. However, often, a surgical birth becomes the next best course of action in a labor, but isn't necessarily a true emergency. Most of the time, cesareans arrive slowly at a birth. I like to say that the shadow of a cesarean walks into a labor room and sits in the corner. Parents may not notice it has entered the room, but most birth professionals do. Usually, that shadow enters long before any conversations are had or any action is taken toward the operating room.

Surgery is an option when labor is not progressing vaginally or when either the birthing parent or baby is not tolerating labor well, and their health is in question. In this way, the need for a birth to occur surgically often builds rather than presenting itself urgently. There are certainly situations where urgency arrives without buildup or warning, but that is definitely not always the case. In the moment of labor when a cesarean enters the conversation, the difference between a true emergency and a non-emergency cesarean can be hard for parents to differentiate, as both can feel surprising and scary.

When a labor starts to show signs that a cesarean delivery might be a good option, that's when parents get to use the B.R.A.I.N. acronym mentioned in chapter 8 along with the other tools for making an informed decision. Involvement in the decision-making process and feeling like the choice was made by *the parents* rather than forced by the provider can help reduce trauma from an unexpected cesarean. When intensity is high, parents often benefit from the support of their birth team. Slowing things down, when possible, is especially helpful in the decision-making process as well as reducing the powerless feelings that can come when things move too fast to fully absorb.

Knowing what happens in a cesarean birth and framing those actions in a helpful context can support parents in navigating an unexpected surgery in a more positive way, and in some cases, reducing trauma.

What Happens in a Cesarean

During an in-labor cesarean, partners are usually separated while each prepares for their unique role in this type of birth. Parents can think of this time as their private time to center and ground themselves for the events to come—especially the arrival of their baby.

Partners are given special paper clothing they wear over their normal clothing. There are pants, a top, shoe coverings, a hairnet, and a surgical mask. These garments are the unique ritualized uniform for a surgical birth. Partners all over the world wear similar items for all cesarean births.

While partners are getting ready, the birthing parent heads into the operating room for their own unique preparation. If they don't already have anesthesia in place, an epidural or a spinal will be inserted. In addition to the medicine to block sensations, there will also be a catheter to empty the bladder and an IV to administer fluids and any additional medications needed. There may also be electrodes to measure heart function, a clip on a fingertip to measure the level of oxygen in the blood, a blood pressure cuff, and for some, an oxygen mask as well. Usually, birthing parents, like their partners, will wear a hairnet as well to protect the surgical opening from stray hairs. To ready the space where the baby will be born, the nursing staff will make sure no pubic hair is in the area by shaving if necessary. They also bathe the area in a rusty red iodine solution. Parents can think of this as a ritual painting of the belly. Many rites of passage involve painting the body as part of the ritual preparation. Often all of the above happens before the birthing parent is reunited with their support person in the operating room.

The lights in an operating room are very bright and the room is usually rather cold. Why is that? The bright lights help to ensure that the specialized team brought together for this birth can see exactly what they are doing. The temperature is kept on the cooler side because it's well known that bacteria grows slower in cold environments, thus aiding the healing process right from the beginning.

It can be surprising for parents to know that the birthing parent's arms are extended out to the sides and often strapped down to boards supporting their arms. Placing the arms out to the sides moves them from the sides of the body where the surgical team needs to be to best do their work. They need to be able to get right up against the body, without obstruction. Parents can request that the arms not be tied down or ask to have the straps left loose, so they act as a reminder not to interfere with the surgical area without being tight.

The other item that is very visible is the drape between the birthing parent's chest and belly. This separates the sterile area from the nonsterile area. Partners and support people can connect with and touch the birthing parent on the nonsterile side of the drape. These drapes are usually blue, but some hospitals now have clear drapes so parents can see the moment of their baby's birth. Some parents grimace when I tell them that watching is occasionally possible. Keep in mind that parents deep into pregnancy can't see their toes when flat on their back; they won't be able to see the incision, which is very low and under the bump of the belly. Where clear drapes are not available, hospital staff will sometimes drop the drape at the time of birth if requested to do so. When the drape is up, the birthing parent has a limited field of vision. As such, it is helpful for the support person to look into the birthing parent's eyes. Since everyone in the room has surgical masks on, the eyes truly become the key mode for visual connection between the partners.

Words are also really helpful. Parents can talk, sing, pray, and express words of love to one another. Their baby is soon to be born!

It can get noisy in a cesarean birth. There may be a lot of talking and activity. Parents who would like it to be quieter can ask the surgical team to limit talking to only what is needed. Some parents say things like, "We'd like to sing a song or welcome our child in silence, so can you limit your conversations please?" Another go-to is to ask for silence to pray. The right to quiet prayer is often respected even when other requests might not be. Some parents prefer to hear the chatter, knowing that if the team is chatting, all is well.

One of the key elements that separates the skills of an obstetrician from that of a midwife is the training and ability to perform a cesarean birth. This is what they have spent years in medical school to be able to do safely. Some parents like to send positive thoughts or blessings to the hands of their surgeon asking them to be steady and skilled during and after the surgery.

Once in the operating room, the moment of birth can happen very quickly but usually takes from fifteen to twenty minutes. When birth is near, there is often a rocking and swaying type of motion as the baby is brought out of the body and into the world. This is a signal that the baby is being born.

Once the baby is out, the surgeon usually displays them over the drape, so the parents can see, but, in most cesarean births I've attended, this is often pretty fast as the baby is taken quickly to the warmer for evaluation to make sure all is well. In cesareans where there isn't concern for the baby and there is a different reason for the baby to be born surgically, then longer connection might be possible.

If skin-to-skin contact, delayed cord clamping, playing music, having other people in the operating room besides just the two parents, or any other special circumstance is important to the family, it is vital to have those conversations ahead of time as part of prenatal preparation for birth. Not all doctors are comfortable accommodating such requests even when parents have asked for them, and knowing that ahead of time can be helpful in determining if the provider's standard of care matches those of the parents.

If the baby is taken to the warmer for evaluation, it is important for the support person to narrate to the birthing parent what is happening. When the baby is out of view, the birthing parent's mind can fill with fantasies about what's happening, and they are rarely positive. The partners or support person can either go over to the warmer and narrate back to the other parent what is happening or can stay at the birthing parent's side and from their vantage point, share what they can see including simple statements like, "They're working hard" or "I see toes!" Some parents go to the warmer and take photos to show the birthing parent. Others don't want their first image of their baby to be on a screen. Birthing parents can decide what feels right for them and share their desires with other members of their birth support team.

At some point, assuming the baby is healthy enough, the newborn is given to the partner to hold (if there is one). Partners tend to hold their newborn the way they would hold the most precious thing ever placed into their arms—carefully and close to their body! This is beautiful but can make it difficult for the birthing parent to see the baby too. Partners need to share the newborn with the birthing parent. They can hold the baby very close to the birthing parent's face so they can kiss, smell, see, and maybe even lick their newborn. We become very primal animals around our newborns so nothing is out of the question in these bonding responses. Other times, birthing parents are not yet back in their bodies themselves and forcing them to "bond" before they are called to naturally can trigger shame that they aren't doing it right. Partners can watch the birthing parent and follow their lead. If they seem to want to connect and start bonding, then partners can bring the newborn close. If they seem to be on a different planet, which is sometimes the case, then partners should wait and let the birthing parent come back into their body first.

After the baby is born, the healing process begins right away. The surgical team will begin to close the opening where the baby was born. This usually takes twenty to forty-five minutes depending on how complex the situation is. During this time, parents can be bonding with their baby or resting.

Once everything is finished in the operating room, the birthing parent is taken to the recovery room to recuperate and to make sure everything is okay before being moved to a postpartum room. During this time, assuming the newborn is healthy, the baby and birthing parent often have a chance to connect, share skin-to-skin contact, and if desired, the birthing parent can initiate breastfeeding. At hospitals that have been designated "Baby Friendly," staff should support birthing parents to be connected with their babies as soon as possible after the birth.[8]

> "Do not expect to be prepared. Life is preparing you to be unprepared. To step from the top of a hundred-foot pole. To have no idea what will happen next. To do whatever is required, without judgment or hesitation." KAREN MAEZEN MILLER[9]

If connecting in the recovery room is not possible due to the health of either baby or parent, then this special bonding time can be delayed until the time when such connection can occur without concern. If that happens, parents can ritualize and redo meeting their baby for the first time.

In addition to reading this section and discussing with your partner anything that came up for you in reading it, I encourage you to have conversations with your medical team about cesarean births. Discuss backup plans with your health-care team. If you're working with a midwife for an out-of-hospital birth, be sure to ask what happens if there is a need to transfer and under what conditions a cesarean would be necessary. Also discuss what important aspects of birth in general can be adapted to a surgical birth such as skin-to-skin contact, delayed cord clamping, cord-blood banking, placenta encapsulation, and so on. Having these conversations prenatally helps address fears and concerns well in advance and in doing so, reduces the unknown factors that tend to feed into sublimated fears.

ONWARD TO BIRTH

You've learned about labor and birth. You've made decisions about your birth and who will be there with you. You've had the conversations you needed to with your partner as well as with your medical team. You've developed and practiced tools for navigating pain and intensity. You've faced the possibility of unexpected and unwanted events becoming a reality. You've practiced facing unexpected and unpredictable experiences. You've dreamed, worked, prayed, learned, softened, strengthened, and loved through the whole process on your way to birth. What is there left to do?

Let go and step bravely across the threshold into the wilderness of birth like an explorer heading into uncharted territory. Carry with you belief in yourself, love for your partner (if you have one), and faith in the process—not that it will follow some idealized image of perfection, but that it will be what it will be *and* that you are courageous and strong enough to face it. You're open, resilient, and strong. And, what's more, you're becoming a parent. On the other side of whatever your birth journey brings is the new world of parenthood.

PART III

On *the* Other Side *of* Birth

It's sadly sort of normal to spend months preparing for birth while forgetting to prepare for what's on the other side. Postpartum preparation, readying for parenthood, and strengthening your relationship for the journey ahead should not be skipped! That's what this part of the book is all about.

The Early Days
of Parenthood

In chapter 4, I shared the labyrinth as a metaphor for labor and birth. When you drew the labyrinth and traced the passage, you found your way to the center—your baby's birth. If the pathway *in* is a metaphor for labor and birth, the path *out* is a metaphor for the journey it takes to come back to yourself, integrated as both a parent *and* an individual.

In my classes, when I ask how long it takes to exit the postpartum labyrinth the most common answers include six weeks (the usual time of the final checkup with your health-care provider), six months, one year, eighteen years, and a lifetime. No answer is wrong as the experience is unique for each person. I believe it is less than a lifetime and far more than six weeks.

I have college-aged kids, and I will say that as much as I feel like I am definitely still on a parenting journey, I don't feel remotely postpartum anymore. The postpartum labyrinth lasts as long as it takes for you to fully integrate your identity as a parent with your nonparent self. This does not happen all at once; nor does it usually take eighteen years. In my case, I only knew once I had *exited* postpartum that I was, in fact, out. I was just exiting my first postpartum labyrinth when I went right back in with the birth of my second child. That labyrinth was very different, but for me, it was also quicker, as the identity transformation was not as uprooting as it had been when I became a mother for the first time.

How long will your journey out of the postpartum labyrinth be? There is no way to know ahead of time.

Some people hear the word *labyrinth* and think of the ancient Greek story of Theseus and the Minotaur. In that story, the beastly Minotaur is trapped in the center of a special labyrinth built by the master builder, Daedalus. Theseus is tasked with entering the labyrinth, killing the Minotaur, and finding his way out again. No one had succeeded before, and Theseus, too, would have failed if not for the support and guidance of an insightful woman, Ariadne, who gives Theseus a ball of thread and tells him to tack one end to the entrance and unroll the thread as he makes his way to the center. Once he has killed the Minotaur, he must follow the thread to make his way out again. While the sound of the beast's roar helps guide Theseus on the way in, coming out is dark and difficult with little to guide him except for that thread.

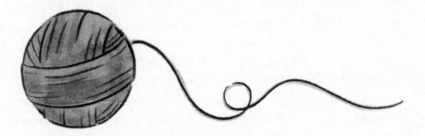

Similarly, the focus on the journey into birth is driven by a clarity of purpose—the birth of your baby—even when faced with doubt or obstacles. The journey out is different. Without a clear destination or definitive direction, the postpartum journey can be cloaked in mystery, doubt, and a feeling of losing your way.

Who or what is your Ariadne?

Preparing early for postpartum—*before* your birth—can profoundly impact your postpartum experience. I encourage parents to have very focused conversations about parenting expectations and to develop strategies for dealing with common challenges ahead of time. This preparatory work is akin to finding your wise guide and gathering the ball of thread, so you can tack it to the threshold and follow it on your way out.

PRENATAL PREPARATION FOR POSTPARTUM

Here are some postpartum topics to discuss and then address before your baby is born.

Practical Support

Postpartum is often a challenging time. You're healing, learning how to parent, and adjusting to life with a baby. Have you thought about how you will get the support you need during that time? Do you have family or friends who can be relied upon to help? What about hiring a postpartum doula if it's affordable? Postpartum doulas are often worth their weight in gold (and doulas-in-training can often be hired at reduced rates). Ask birth doulas in your area for recommendations or go online to one of the many doula registries.

Emotional Well-Being

Think about ways you can support yourself emotionally and how those around you can help. What is your "water of life" or the emotional sustenance that will help you become vibrant again?

Who will be your parenting community? Find or make your village! This is likely the number one suggestion I have for individuals heading into parenthood. Learn where other new parents gather, such as at baby groups, mother's groups, mommy/daddy-and-me exercise classes, working mother's groups, stay-at-home father's groups, LGBTQ parent groups, parenting philosophy/education groups, such as Resources for Infant Educarers (or RIE) classes and attachment parenting, community meetups for walks or visits to parks, zoos, and other public areas, lactation groups (like La Leche League), and so on.

What about other ways to support your postpartum period that you can enjoy from your home without any need to venture out? I recommend finding books to read or podcasts or audiobooks to listen to that support your emotional, intellectual, or spiritual well-being. Similarly, find online groups or resources that support new parents like Facebook groups and Instagram accounts with inspiring content (look for accounts that address the truth of both the joys and the challenges). Aim for inspiration not perfection. Sometimes accounts that focus on beauty or lifestyle can be triggering in postpartum rather than supportive. Find the people who are speaking the truth about the challenges and thriving anyway.

Household Chores

After the baby's born, how will household tasks such as cooking, cleaning, grocery shopping, and laundry get done and to what level of completeness? What are your expectations about how clean your home will be after your baby arrives? How often is the laundry done and to what level of completeness: hung to dry or in the dryer, clean in a laundry basket or folded and put away?

What about food? How freshly cooked do your meals need to be? How often will groceries fill your cupboards and fridge? It can be really helpful to plan, prepare, and freeze meals ahead of time for the early postpartum period. Or ask a close friend to organize a meal train to have loved ones bring you food after your baby arrives.[2]

Baby Care

How will the needs of your baby be met? Who will care for your baby during the night? How about during the day? What part will be shared, what part will be taken care of exclusively by one parent or by someone else? If other people will be involved in your child's care, how will that person be found/hired? Who will make those arrangements?

What about diapers? Will you go with disposables, a cloth diaper delivery service, or cloth diapers washed at home? Or perhaps you're planning to use no diapers at all and practice elimination communication. What more do you need to know to implement the system you want to use once baby is here?

How will you feed your baby? If you plan to breastfeed, who will support your learning process? Can you familiarize yourself with helpful resources in your area? La Leche League meetings are free and often a good place to learn about breastfeeding, or you might engage a lactation specialist. As much as possible, make these arrangements before your baby arrives, while your level of energy and independence are higher. Breastfeeding can be hard and facing challenges with tools can be very helpful.

Take a baby care class and infant CPR, especially if you have little or no experience with newborns or want to learn more. You will also need to select a pediatrician.

Parenting Styles

How do you want to parent? How might you share decision-making responsibilities—equally, or allowing the parent who does more of the caregiving to have a greater voice, or something else? How will you figure out what is best for your baby? How will you handle disagreements about parenting styles? Who are your go-to parenting guides—friends, family, books, or experts?

Try reading a parenting book or two alone or with your partner before your baby is born to begin developing a vision of how you would like to parent. Even if you don't like what's in the book, you'll learn a lot by reading it. My website (brittabushnell.com/resources) has a list of suggested titles you can start with.

Sleep

What about sleep? I'm talking about yours here, not the baby's. Prepare for the very real possibility that you will have broken sleep for many months, and while this is normal, it can be exhausting. It is *unusual* for babies to sleep more than a few hours at a stretch for the first four to six months. What strategies do you imagine using to help you navigate this part of the postpartum experience together? Who is available to help you—family, friends, or paid support? The number one thing new parents need to heal from birth is rest. Brainstorm ideas now about how to get more rest when you need it.

Postpartum Mood Disorders

It's a good idea to learn the symptoms and signs of postpartum depression, anxiety, PTSD, and postnatal psychosis, as well as other common mood disorders and where you can get help if any of these arise in postpartum.[3] If you already have a relationship with a trusted healing professional—whether it's a therapist, psychiatrist, life coach, chiropractor, spiritual or religious guide, or mentor—maintain contact with them. This doesn't necessarily have to be someone you pay—a friend or elder in your life whose support you appreciate can work just as well. Sometimes postpartum mood disorders require help from a professional specifically trained in treating them.

I know that preparing for the postpartum period can feel like just another thing to do on an already long to-do list to prepare for birth! Still, I encourage you to spend at least as much time preparing for postpartum as you do for labor and birth.[1] Let's face it, postpartum is a lot longer and, for many, far harder than labor and birth. When you feel lost, what you have researched and put in place prenatally will be there to help you find your way through.

While exploring the areas mentioned above can be helpful as you prepare for postpartum, remember that control, certainty, and perfection are unattainable, as they are illusions. Postpartum is still a wild, unpredictable time of transformation. The cultural ideals addressed in part 2 permeate postpartum too. Like birth, postpartum is an unknowable experience that requires maturity, flexibility, resilience, and courage.

WELCOME TO PARENTHOOD!

Congratulations on the birth of your baby! You're a parent now. Holy shit . . . it really did happen! Yep. Now, the next chapter of your life begins in earnest.

The Center of the Labyrinth

You've given birth. Like Theseus, you did what you came to do. Now what? First, allow yourself to be in the center of your journey—to pause, to stop, to wait, to listen, and to rest. The center is a powerful place in itself. Do not rush the journey of healing, processing, and returning. Transformation is often a slow and messy process.

This very early part of postpartum, sometimes defined as the first six weeks or the first forty days, is a highly sensitive and important part of the first three months of new parenthood. In terms of the labyrinth metaphor, these days are the center and maybe the first few steps outward. Here, progress on your journey back to yourself is rarely obvious. At this time, you really aren't moving forward toward your former self; instead, you're letting the transformation into parenthood unfold.

Take the first step only when you are ready to begin. Like the journey into the labyrinth, the journey out happens one step at a time. In the beginning of your journey out, everything seems to circle around the birth and the baby. It can feel like your former identity is a very, very long way off, and indeed, the goal is not to return to your former identity but to create your new one that *includes* parenthood. You may not recognize yourself at all—feeling instead like someone who *only* has a baby or who has just given birth. It can feel like there is no other part of you. In many ways, all there is in those early days is a newborn baby and newborn parents. This period of time can be clunky and emotional. Each step forward feels like it comes with two steps backward. But like the journey toward birth, the main things you have to do to get out of the labyrinth are keep going and stay in the moment rather than getting ahead of yourself.

No One Ever Told Me

One of the things I hear frequently from new parents is the phrase, "No one ever told me." What varies in these statements is the thing they've never been told. Just as in birth, new parenthood comes with unexpected surprises, both welcome and unwelcome.

One new mother, Katherine, shared her version of "no one ever told me" on social media: "I wish I had not been told over and again that "it's worth it." I expected the hardship to come, but didn't expect the exhaustion that would feel like I couldn't do it anymore and that there had to be a different better way that no one had shared with me. I thought no one understood because some days it really didn't feel "worth it." How could the destruction of me be good and healthy for my child? I wish someone had said, "You will doubt yourself. You will feel lost. You will wonder if it was worth it. In the end, you will find a new you and a path you didn't know existed."

Just as the labyrinthine journey into birth twists and turns in ways that seem to take you away from your intended destination, so, too, does the journey out. You will face unexpected events, emotions, and challenges. Exactly what they will be, no one can tell you ahead of time. Surprises are an inherent part of the experience. Familiarizing yourself with what typically happens in early parenthood can be helpful, but knowing there will be unexpected trials, no matter how much you've prepared, is even more important.

Lifestyle Adjustments and the First Forty Days

For many new parents, there are major, often challenging, adjustments to their lifestyle after the arrival of a newborn. Before giving birth, even deep into pregnancy, you have a high degree of autonomy, independence, and flexibility in the flow of your life. In the first few weeks after birth, life pretty much occurs at the whim and mercy of your child.

While this is normal, it's almost never easy. Days and nights are loaded with all things baby. This nurturing fills your time, leaving very little space to do anything else or put attention on anyone else. These days can feel frustrating for those parents used to doing a lot, working long hours, engaging with other adults, pursuing a daily exercise or personal practice, or following other desires or hobbies. This phase can look and feel like "doing nothing." But this is far from the truth. Even though it might look like you're not doing anything "productive," you are doing critical work nurturing your baby and healing yourself. Slowing down and changing your definition of productivity is essential in new parenthood. Also remember this period is temporary and will gradually change over time.

Lying-In

In many cultures around the world, this period of time is honored as a time when a new parent isn't expected to do anything beyond healing and resting—they practice "lying in." Other people, often extended family, cook and feed the new parent as well as the other members of the household. They do the laundry, of which there is so much (how does such a tiny human make so much dirty laundry?). They clean your home and help with the baby so that you can get the rest you desperately need. In some cultures, postpartum parents observe a period of confinement where they do not leave the home or, in some cases, even their bedroom, for a number of weeks. They cocoon themselves in a physical way that mirrors the cocooning process going on internally.

In Latin America this time is known as *la cuarentena*, which literally means "quarantine." Some form of a lying-in period is practiced in Indonesia, Malaysia, Korea, India, Zambia, Egypt, Japan, China, and among Native American tribes.[4] It is not a common practice in most Western countries, but it is catching on as those raised where postpartum care practices and rituals are respected, share their wisdom. *The First Forty Days* by Heng Ou is a beautiful book about this practice.

I love the *idea* of a lying-in period for all new families. I have had clients rave about the experience. I think it is important, however, to remember that most Western cultures have not integrated this type of support into postpartum care. Frankly, postpartum care is nearly nonexistent in the United States and many other Western countries. By contrast, new Dutch mothers are given an in-home support person paid for by the government. I love this idea so much! Unfortunately, the practices of lying-in and of receiving regular emotional and practical help from others are not the norm for most postpartum families. That means if you want it, you will likely have to hire a postpartum doula, ask a close relative to come stay with you, rally your community of loved ones to participate in a rotating schedule of support, or set up food delivery as well as household help. It also means that if you try a lying-in period and it doesn't work for you, the reasons could be cultural rather than personal.

Remember that you may *want* to do a special lying-in period and still find when you get to that point that some aspects of lying-in just don't feel right. It is important to hold all of your prenatal ideas about what will help you during postpartum without attachment as things can and often do change. Some parents need to get out of the house for their emotional well-being. Some do best staying home. Pay attention to what works for you, not what works for your friend or sister, not what you read about in a book or heard about on a podcast. Listen to what your psyche needs and respond as best you can to what it tells you.

Extended Family

Exploring the lying-in period usually brings me to the topic of extended family. If your parents and/or your partner's parents are still alive, chances are you're having conversations about what happens after the birth of your baby. And when parents are becoming grandparents for the first time, the intensity is generally heightened. Complex shifts are underway as children become parents and parents become grandparents. As you birth yourself into parenthood, huge tectonic shifts occur in the bedrock of your relationship with *your* parents. Your relationship with each other has developed over years and decades—solidifying your roles as parent and child. They are used to being the parent with all that that involves, including decision-making rights over parenting styles.

Identity transformation happens on all fronts. This transition turns the archetypal wheel of a family, reorienting who falls into each identity—your baby becomes the child, you become the parent, your new family becomes the family, and your parents become the grandparents.

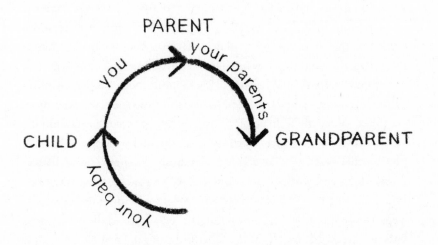

This is big, and it's often disorienting while the shift happens and new roles settle into place. It is normal for this reorientation to cause friction, upset, and conflict. It is unfamiliar territory for everyone involved, and no one yet knows how to behave toward and around each other in their new identity.

Setting boundaries that support your new family is a huge and sometimes difficult part of new parenthood. Doing so helps everyone shift into their new identity on the family wheel, including *you*, and also helps establish which relationships are primary. New parents can feel overwhelmed and unsettled by having to tell their parents—the new grandparents—what is and isn't allowed. As difficult as these conversations can be at times, they're part of the maturation process necessary in parenthood. It's common for the gears to grind at first as the archetypal wheel turns.

This change in decision-making power extends to parenting styles. As the parents, it's your choice whether or not you accept the opinions, advice, or guidance from the new grandparents, and it's also your right to ask them to withhold certain opinions or judgments that you don't want to hear. It's normal to reflect on your own upbringing and what you would like to keep and change about the way you were raised, while at the same time exploring new parenting concepts and learning new information that may not have been available to your parents when they were raising you. Sometimes, it isn't a matter of style, but one of memory!

When my little sister gave birth for the first time, my stepmom balked at the new mom's insistence that everyone wash their hands carefully before holding my newborn nephew. My stepmom, who had successfully raised six of her own kids to adulthood, had the memory of the cleanliness standards she kept by the time she had given birth six times! What she didn't consciously remember were her cleanliness standards when *she* was a first-time mom. Since I was eight when my first brother was born, and I had very limited experience with newborns, the green bottles of antibacterial soap in each bathroom of our home that *everyone* was instructed to use before holding the new baby, were highly memorable! I know for me, even after only having two kids, my standards for cleanliness changed from my first to my second. Imagine having six! Hers was a perspective borne from having many children and as a result, she could hardly relate to the caution and protectiveness exhibited by a first-time parent.

No parenting is perfect since perfection is an unattainable illusion. But it is your right to do the best job you can according to what you and your partner think is best. What's more, you have the right to screw up parenting in your own unique way. In fact, you *will* screw it up in your own way. You get to make mistakes just like your parents did. Everyone makes mistakes in parenting. Even if you do the absolute best job you can, there will be times when you or your children reflect back on their childhood and wish you had done something differently. What's more, remember that it is not your responsibility to make other people, including family, comfortable with your parenting decisions.

Remember the exercise of building a bridge from chapter 8? With extended family, practice building a bridge of shared positive intention whenever possible. Listen to the positive intention beneath their strategy or suggestion. Speak it back to them and check it out. Let's say your mom makes a negative comment about sleeping with your baby and co-sleeping has been your go-to sanity saver. Start building a bridge by mirroring her positive intention and then get curious. This might sound something like, "You're worried about the welfare of our baby and are concerned that co-sleeping might not be what's best for him. Is that right?" Stick with the place where you meet: concern for the welfare of your baby. You might have differing *strategies* for addressing that concern, but it is helpful to meet in the place where you share a common purpose. Battles focused entirely on conflicting strategies are rarely productive.

Through all the highs and lows with extended family, remember that new grandparents are going through an identity transformation as well. As much as possible, give them space to change and adjust, just as you desire the same from them. Still, when needed, hold your boundaries and parent in way that is best suited to you, your family, and your values.

POSTPARTUM HEALING

In addition to adjusting to parenting a newborn, you're also healing from the birth process. This should not be underestimated. Your body is changing more in a few days than it ever has in your lifetime. This hormonal shift is guiding your body from a pregnant state to a post-pregnancy state of bonding and/or lactating. We'll address this hormonal shift more in chapter 13.

Physical Healing

There are also physical wounds from pregnancy and birth that need time to heal. In addition to vaginal or perineal stitches, a cesarean incision, or vaginal stretching and other visible wounds, there is also the *invisible* wound in your uterus. When the placenta separates, it leaves an open wound about the size of a salad plate where it had been connected and merged with the lining of your uterus. This raw opening has to close and heal while the uterus shrinks back to its pre-pregnancy size, which takes time and rest. In the first week after birth, your uterus shrinks to half of its immediate post-birth size. By four weeks postpartum, it will be back to about its pre-pregnancy size.

During this process, called "involution," the uterus sluffs its lining in what can be like a very heavy period, which usually lasts from two to six weeks after birth. The blood flow is heaviest during the first week or so after birth, but then it slows and you can use it as an indicator of when you're doing too much. If your flow has slowed overall and then picks up again after you go out and run errands, chances are your body is letting you know that your level of activity was too much, too soon.

My second baby was born in the middle of October, and his older brother was two and a half at the time, just old enough to be very excited by the idea of Halloween. We lived in a very hilly rural neighborhood where houses were pretty far apart. Trick-or-treating in our town closely resembled hiking at night in costume! I didn't want to miss taking part in it with my wide-eyed toddler, so I strapped our two-week-old to my body and headed out for this fall ritual. About halfway through our small neighborhood, I realized I had taken on too much. I started bleeding heavily and turned on my heels and headed home. My body was letting me know that it was too early for hiking even if I called it trick-or-treating!

Postpartum is a time for rest, even if you feel great. The reconfiguration going on in your physical body is profound. Some new parents feel a surge of energy in early postpartum and a readiness to charge toward the exit of the labyrinth. If you experience this, exercise caution and reenter your physical life slowly. I have heard numerous stories of new parents who start exercising or exerting themselves physically before their body has healed from the momentous experience of birth. The best early postpartum exercise is to practice patience. Take it slowly. (I recommend reading Kimberly Ann Johnson's *The Fourth Trimester* for more specific guidance.)

Emotional Healing

Giving birth is a huge experience and one that often requires time and care to heal and move through your emotional body. Some births don't need much attention at all, while others need intensive and intentional effort to process.

Processing Your Birth Experience

One of the tendencies after a powerful experience is self-judgment fueled by hindsight. A coach I worked with called these COWS, which stood for "could, ought, would, should."[5] These are the voices that berate us for not doing something *then* that we can imagine doing *now*: "I could have . . . ," "I ought to have . . . ," "If only I would have . . . ," or "I should have . . . " These inquiries don't help and usually make the healing process more painful. And what's more, COWS are full of bullshit! Hindsight judgment has a way of replaying situations and believing that we could have done something differently to alter the events in a more positive direction. You did the very best you could in that moment, and if you *could* have done something differently, you would have.

During experiences of heightened emotion, such as birth, we don't have access to all of our regular responses. We need to understand how the body works in response to a threat. Trauma expert Peter Levine says of this state:

> Without access to normal orienting responses, when threatened we are unable to successfully escape even when the situation offers that possibility. We may not even see it. Arousal is so strongly linked with immobility that the two can't be separated. Arousal leads to immobility. Period. Any time we are aroused, we automatically feel immobilized and helpless. And we are. We may be fortified by adrenaline and physically able to run, but the sense of helplessness is so strong that we are unable to find the exit and leave.[6]

Sometimes, you can't act, even when you want to. Using your normal orienting responses against yourself after the fact doesn't take into consideration all of the factors influencing your action or inaction in the moment. The answer to "Why didn't I?" is often that you couldn't.

The tendency after birth is to either share or keep secret your birth story. Neither is a completely healthy way to process the rite of passage of birth. When we share our story over and over again, the story becomes more real than the experience itself. The story of what happened becomes our experience, and unhooking from that story can be difficult when we've laid the track of it over and over again through the retelling, without fresh insight or recognition of nuanced details. When we tell our traumatic story over and over believing it's cathartic to do so or hoping repetition will help us work through it, we can unintentionally reinforce a false belief that memory is completely truthful (which it isn't) and accidentally fortify the trauma.[7]

Healing is not a linear process. There is no one way to heal or an easy-to-follow trajectory for healing. Emotional repair is a labyrinthine journey all its own. You may feel better one day and find yourself in the depths of struggle again the next. This is normal, but you do not have to face it alone. Seek out help from a therapist, somatic healer, a loving friend, or someone trained as a Birth Story Listener.[8]

You can also begin to process the experience on your own. Most important is to allow the feelings that arise to be felt. Shutting down genuine emotions because you or someone else thinks they are inappropriate, irrational, or too big suppresses the healing process, making it harder to move through. Give yourself space to feel your feelings . . . all of them. This can be confusing when you have a beloved baby in your arms and simultaneously feel grief, rage, or despair. Make space for whatever emotion comes without judgment. What helps you access and feel your emotions? For many, journaling, art, exercise, or being in nature can help. Let the healing process move at its own pace. You can't get there all at once. Be patient and move out of the labyrinth one small step at a time.

> "Grief, fear, and despair are primary human emotions. Without them, we would be less than human, and less likely to survive. Grief arises because we are not alone, and what connects us to others and to the world also breaks our hearts. Grieving our losses allows us to heal and renew our spirits. Fear alerts us to protect our survival, extending beyond our instinct for self-preservation to our concern for others. Despair asks us to find meaning in the midst of apparent chaos or meaninglessness. Making meaning out of suffering is the basis of the human capacity to survive evil and transcend it." MIRIAM GREENSPAN[9]

Heightened Sensitivity

It's normal to have heightened sensitivity during postpartum. This tenderness comes from hormones and the raw-heartedness that often comes along with new parenthood. Things matter and touch us in ways we may never have experienced before. This is not being irrational or hysterical. It's the vulnerability and tenderness of new parenthood, and as such deserves our respect rather than scorn. Instead of belittling these new emotional sensitivities, attend to them and listen to what they need from you. Respect this tenderness rather than degrade it as some sort of failure.

I found in early parenthood that I had to stop listening to the news and change the types of movies and shows I watched. After the birth of my first baby, I was porous like a sponge. Everything that came in through my ears or eyes went directly to my heart. Violence, heart-wrenching tragedy, emotional trauma—I just couldn't handle any of it. This type of sensitivity can extend to social media, TV shows, and even to people around you. During postpartum, it's as if your nerves are raw and bare. Give yourself permission to protect yourself from unnecessary intensity. Remember, you're in a cocoon reforming yourself, and your nervous system is exposed. Since you can't spin an actual cocoon of silk around yourself, you need to protect your tender metamorphic process in other ways.

This heightened sensitivity is also highly susceptible to the pit of comparison. Be careful with the tendency to compare yourself to others—in real life, online, or in the media. The inclination to be hard on yourself is likely elevated. Work to keep yourself in the moment—this moment, right here, right now. That's it. The seven tips I share in the next chapter will help with this too.

STILL IN THE WILDERNESS

Remember Artemis from chapter 5? She's not done with you yet. Just because you've given birth doesn't mean you've left Artemis's wilderness. Birth and postpartum are a wild landscape not just because they are unfamiliar and nature based, but also because they exist in a place between worlds. It is an unfamiliar wilderness. Psychiatrist and author Jean Shinoda Bolen says this about Artemis's wilderness, and it pertains to postpartum beautifully:

> Wilderness is a metaphoric landscape; it is where you are in your life when you are in between one major phase or

identity and the next. It's a time to make your own way, when you do not know what will come next or how you will change. It is a time of transition. It may be a time to trust instinct or deep curiosity. You may find an important part of yourself in this wilderness, or lose your bearings and become lost. . . . You are in the wilderness when you have left "who" you were, and there is no turning back.[9]

Like labor, postpartum is still Artemisian—it's unpredictable, wild, unstructured, tied to the cycles of nature, private, earthy, chaotic, connected to the animal nature of your own body, often lonely, and most importantly, untamed. It is precisely this hazier, less-structured quality of the childbearing period that defines time in both labor and new parenthood. It is not connected to productivity and output.

While experiencing cyclical time might be a gift of pregnancy, childbirth, and lactation, most of the pregnant people who come through my classes express frustration at this unfamiliar, messy, and unstructured time.

"The woman has survived the ordeal of the underworld and returned from that dark abode to ordinary life. She bears now the marks of the initiation on the inner chambers of her soul where Ereshkigal sits heavily upon her throne. Life in the upper world goes on as before. No one may notice the change in her at all." BETTY DE SHONG MEADOR[11]

The lack of familiarity is part of the process. You don't need to know everything ahead of time. No one ever goes into the wilderness knowing ahead of time what they will encounter. You prepare for what you can and gather your courage, resilience, and fortitude to face the unexpected. Just as the exercises, myths, and metaphors from the previous chapters supported you to face the unexpected in birth, they are useful in postpartum too. Ascending from an experience of the Underworld involves facing gates and challenges as you slowly climb your way back to the surface.

Transformed Parenthood

There is becoming a parent and there is learning to parent. These are two separate but connected parts of the postpartum experience. One relates to identity and the other to skill development. For a while, they grow in tandem—one along with the other, learning skills while you get to know yourself as a parent. At some point, you realize your identity transformation has more or less happened—you know yourself as a parent. But developing parenting skills is a multidecade endeavor that is ever evolving. My kids are nineteen and sixteen as I write this. My identity as their mother has been well-established for many years, but I am constantly learning how to parent each of them as the situation and phase changes.

NURTURING THE PARENT IN YOU

For years I have said in my classes that parents are only as old as their baby. When a baby is one hour old, the parent is a one-hour-old parent. When a baby is a week old, the parents are also only a week old. Parents don't scold their baby to stand up and run when they are just learning to crawl. Even if running is a far more efficient way to get around, we understand the developmental stages and changes a baby needs to go through to progress. Parents know babies need to go through many stages before they are able to run. We wouldn't think of berating a child for not knowing how to do something before its time. And yet, as parents, we do this to ourselves all the time. For some reason, when a baby is born, parents often expect themselves to know all the ins and outs of parenting before their baby is a week old! A lot of energy is spent judging and criticizing ourselves for *learning* how to parent, believing instead that we should just innately know how to do it!

Perhaps these unreasonable expectations we place on ourselves are due to how high the stakes feel when we are learning how to care for our new child. We feel we have to know how to do this or else. This attitude, coupled with the cultural ideals of perfection and independence, makes learning to parent both extra challenging and an opportunity for profound personal growth.

Parenting Is Like Cooking

Learning how to parent is like learning how to cook. You start out learning from your parents or other cooks around you, then you might take a class or two and buy a cookbook and other kitchen tools, but at some point, to really learn how to cook, you have to do it. Even the best cooks have dishes that flop, especially if they're putting themselves out there and trying new things. As you keep practicing in the kitchen, you get better. The cookbooks and online recipes are likely still there when you need them, but over time, you develop your own style of cooking.

This is just like learning to parent. You've learned about parenting throughout your lifetime from those who raised you, elders, and even peers on the parenting path ahead of you. You might take parenting classes in newborn care, breastfeeding, or sleep, or study a specific parenting philosophy.

Then there are the parenting books! My library of parenting books actually surpasses my library of cookbooks. Like my cookbooks, I haven't read every parenting book cover to cover, but I know where to look when I need help with a specific parenting challenge, just like I consult a cookbook when I can't remember the ratio of broth to rice when making risotto in my pressure cooker (something I can never seem to remember even though I cook it often). And, like my cookbooks, some of my parenting books sit neglected while others are dog-eared, with tabbed pages, underlined passages, and well-used sections that open automatically.

What parents need to remember is to use parenting books and experts the way cookbooks and cooking classes are intended: to help you develop your own unique style. There are times in parenting, like in cooking (baking especially), when following a proven recipe helps make the situation's end result better. For some, these include feeding routines and practices, sleep methods, following unique protocols for kids with special needs, and more. Even when following prescribed formulas for specific tasks, make sure to keep your heart and gut engaged so you can *feel* if what you're trying is right for *you*.

Feed Your Curiosity and Bolster Your Intuition

New parents are often told to "listen to their intuition." While this advice is a nice idea, it isn't enough and often leaves new parents adrift wondering where their illusive "intuition" is located in the first place! For parents steeped in a culture where oceans of information are available at our fingertips, listening to an inner voice of guidance is rarely a honed skill. Additionally, the intuitive voice rarely sounds certain and, as a result, is often dismissed.

To begin bolstering your intuitive voice, start by renaming it "curiosity." Being curious is often how the intuitive voice first whispers in your ear. Activate your curiosity and then pause before you feed the curiosity what it's hungry for.

How do you feed your curiosity and help develop a louder intuitive voice? Before you begin to cook a meal or even look in a cookbook for a recipe, you have to ask yourself the question, "What am I hungry for?" Similarly, listening to your intuition starts by asking yourself, "What do I need to know?" As discussed in chapter 4, insert a much-needed pause between curiosity's question and taking action to find answers *out there*.

Research has shown that it can be difficult to activate curiosity without a baseline of information since without any information or experience on a topic, we don't even have the awareness to know what we don't know.[1] Curiosity thrives on being fed *enough* information. And new experiences make us aware of what we don't know. This is why new situations, like becoming a parent for the first time, evoke a lot of curiosity.

Develop a baseline of information in parenting by observing others, reading books, listening to podcasts, or taking classes, whatever brings you into contact with ideas about parenting. It's difficult to consult your intuition about a topic you know nothing about. Once you've fed your curiosity, you must inquire within yourself if what you've seen, read, or heard works for you and your family. In this way, intuition is a way of processing information you've gathered, experiences you've had, thoughts you've pondered, questions you've asked, and unfamiliar territories you've explored. It isn't a single inner voice that you simply have to listen to; it is the processor itself.

Facing Opposing Voices

One of the most challenging parts of new parenthood is navigating the sea of opinions *out there* and weeding through them all to discover what's true for you and your baby. What adds to this challenge is that some of those external voices and opinions come from supposed experts.

I remember when I was a brand-new mom, I dutifully took my son to all the pediatrician appointments "on schedule." At each appointment I brought up my concerns and questions as well as my thoughts regarding these concerns and questions. Our doctor had his spiel for the six-week, three-month, and six-month checkups. To me, it felt like he was on rote, delivering his message depending on the age of my son, not based on what I was bringing to the appointment. My son's pediatrician was an expert on babies, and I was a first-time mom. At first, I would attentively listen to every word believing I was learning from a master. But over time, I began to realize that while he might be an expert on babies generally, I was the expert regarding *my* baby.

As I began to feel my mother legs solidifying beneath me, I started interrupting the doctor and being more assertive about asking my questions and getting my needs met. Before my son turned one, I found a new doctor.

What might surprise you is that I am profoundly grateful for the months I spent under the care of our family's first pediatrician. He gave me what I needed in those early months when I believed I needed to be told what I should do with my child. He provided exactly what I thought I needed. It was only later that I found I needed something else. It was under his care that I developed the courage to change my mind simply because I wanted a different type of relationship with my son's doctor. What I needed as a parent of a newborn was different from what I needed as a parent of an eight-month-old.

Letting your parenting legs develop and support you will likely take time. As you grow as a parent, you might find that advice and guidance from books, experts, and guides of all sorts no longer suit you, even if they did early on. Let yourself be fluid in your decisions. Allow your mind to change *and let that be okay.* Do not judge yourself now for what you didn't know or didn't care about *back then.* Your needs and values grow with you as you evolve as a parent.

Small Steps

It's typical for parents to notice what's broken or not working in our parenting. This has to do in part with the quest for perfection I addressed in chapter 10. When we measure or even just take notice of how we're doing, we tend to focus on the lack—the space between where we think we are and where we think we *should be.* This is a problem-focused mind-set where attention is given to the problem or gap between what is currently true and where we want to be in the future. Instead, try the following exercise.

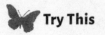 **Try This**

Making It Just a Little Bit Better

Go through the following questions and take your time answering each one. I recommend journaling as you do so.

- What would you like to be different about your parenting?

- Suppose you felt the way you'd like to about your parenting:
  - » What would be different?
  - » How would you know it was different?
  - » In a future place where this is already different, how did you help make it happen?

- Imagine a scale of one to ten, where ten is you feeling the way you want to about your parenting day in and day out without ever slipping or having any bad moments, and one is the worst you can possibly imagine. Where on the scale is your parenting today?
  - » Why is your parenting there and not *lower*?
  - » How come it's that high?
  - » Notice all the things you're doing that are already okay or don't suck.

- Now imagine it's a week from now and your parenting is getting just a little bit better.
  - » What would be different that would let you know that your parenting is getting better?
  - » Who would notice it was getting better?

- What's one small step you could take in the next twenty-four hours that would improve the chances of parenting getting just a little bit better?[2]

It can be overwhelming to try to improve and make things better when times are really hard. Small steps make a big difference. Don't expect yourself to be a ten on the scale. That's aiming for perfect, and perfect is overrated. Aim for feeling good about what you're doing and how you're doing it . . . much of the time. There will always be times when we fall off our parenting horse. Your job is not to be a flawless rider but to be able to climb back on when you get knocked off. You will get knocked around in the arena of parenthood. That's the nature of the job! Rather than aiming for perfect, aim for good enough and slowly feeling more grounded as a parent, even in the moments you're thrown off center.

Family Rituals

Along the path of parenthood, you will be weaving the threads for what will likely become a rich tapestry of family rituals and traditions that help to define what is meant by "family" beyond what is biological or legal. Families thrive on rituals because rituals tell us who we are as a group of people knit together beyond the bonds of love. Note that if you don't consciously create family rituals, they will be created without your awareness, and you might not like them!

What's more is that people—babies and children in particular—respond positively to regularity, predictability, and rhythms in their day, week, and year. Before babies are able to tell time, they begin to respond to the nightly rituals involved with bedtime. Long before children can read or understand a calendar, they learn to appreciate seasonal and holiday traditions.

As you begin to settle into your life as parents, pay attention to the parts of your daily life that form rituals. Weave them throughout your day and your child's day. When you wake up, you do this, and when it's time for bed, you do that. Babies respond to the repetition and the ritualization and even come to expect it. This can make your life easier. Bedtime becomes a rhythmic dance with specialized steps toward sleep. Use rituals to embed your family's values into your daily habits or routines. Over time, these will grow and shift as you move through the years, but from my experience, they give both structure and beauty to the family tapestry.

The Myth of Self-Care and
How to Really Tend to Your Soul[3]

I often hear new parents, especially new mothers, talk about the importance of self-care. Birth professionals also drive home the need for new parents to take care of themselves. And while I agree it is important to take care of yourself while caring for a child, be careful not to use this idea against yourself as one more way you aren't "measuring up."

When our first child, Kaden, was born, my husband and I lived in a studio guest house. We cooked, ate, slept, worked, and socialized all in the same one room. For the first several days after Kaden was born, even my mom shared that living space with us. Privacy wasn't just a privilege; it was an unattainable illusion! Even though that baby is now in college, I remember those early days well. Each day was a process of going from diaper change to feeding and back again. In some ways, that one room made things simpler if not easier. The world my little family and I created was contained within one set of walls. The act of going from bed to kitchen involved not much more than a roll out of bed followed by a few steps or stumbles.

When Kaden was a few months old, we moved into our home. Suddenly, we had closing doors and the possibility of privacy, our baby had a room of his own, and we finally had a closet! And while the space brought breathing room for all of us, it also added to my list of things to "get done." When wrapped in the womb of that small one-room studio, we stumbled around those precious and difficult postpartum days without many expectations. Nothing beyond caring for our new amazing family member held much importance. The rub really started after we moved, after our baby was less freshly born, and after I really started to believe, "I got this."

It was at that point when I began believing I could get shit done—dishes, the laundry, the toilets, the yard, the garbage, family gatherings, and my work. The to-do list grew along with my competence, keeping relaxation forever slightly out of reach. Around this time, I began hearing the mantra of self-care. Now, in addition to everything else on my to-do list, I also had to make sure I "took care of myself."

Instead of helping a new parent actually tend to themselves, the rally cry for self-care can make parents weary, increasing the list of things they can't seem to get done! Many of us want to adopt new self-care practices and rituals—meditation, yoga, journaling—and when we don't keep them going or find that the job of parenting always seems to get in the way, we collapse upon our own best intentions. A teacher of mine once said to me, "We cannot force ourselves into a new spiritual or self-care practice. We must be called to it from joy rather than obligation."[4]

What calls to you from joy? What calls you to tend to it not because you should, but because the whispering voice in your belly yearns to be heard? Move toward that longing with small movements—not as another thing to check off your to-do list but rather as a momentary gift to your soul. It may be as simple as a few present moments in the shower while you feel the warm water roll down your skin, and the aroma of a favorite soap fills your senses.

Self-care can be made up of small moments rather than grand gestures. Think of self-care as a moment of remembering to be in your own body. Notice what you are feeling, breathe a deeper breath, and inhale a smell you enjoy—one that reminds you that being human isn't all about baby poop and spit-up. Self-care doesn't necessarily require a babysitter or even time alone. It can simply be opening yourself to your own bodily experience and turning toward a moment of enjoyment. I invite you to make a ritual of turning toward yourself as a regular practice beyond the list of self-care activities adorning social media. Candles are not required.

THE PROFOUND PRACTICE OF PARENTING

Sure, birth is a transformative experience ripe with opportunities for spiritual and personal growth—that makes sense. You got that, right? But the opportunities for inner growth don't end the moment the baby arrives. Quite the opposite! Parenthood is a path that will test you at every turn and provide you with unending opportunities to evolve as a person. Parenting, like practices such as mindfulness, yoga, contemplative prayer, creative expression, or other similar endeavors, requires great focus, pushes you to your edge of comfort, forces you to grow and makes you do all of that over again day after day. In this way, the path of parenthood is a profound personal practice.

Most of what parents need during the journey of parenthood exists within their own minds. Let's face it, part of what makes parenting such an intense personal growth path is that it is wildly difficult to escape it. Even when your kids are not around you, their presence lingers in your heart. Here are seven reminders to help you on the profound path of parenting. The sections that follow provide more detail for each reminder.

1. Cut yourself some slack.

2. Practice self-forgiveness.

3. Stay in the moment.

4. Expand your expectations.

5. Soften your attachments.

6. Ask for and accept help.

7. Nurture a kind inner voice.

Cut Yourself Some Slack

Parenting is nothing if not a brutal practice in humility! No one is capable of perfection in parenting . . . and anyone who believes such a thing exists either hasn't had kids or is fooling themselves. Expect to make mistakes. Nearly every parent has *many* moments when they suck at parenting or just can't seem to get it. Early on there are the moments when we can't seem to figure out how to soothe an inconsolable baby or we put on a diaper that slips off as soon as we pick up our baby.

I remember the time my firstborn rolled off the bed when I didn't expect it and landed unharmed but wailing on the floor. And the time I fastened his diaper so tightly that when I took it off a few hours later he had red lines where the diaper had been cutting into his tender skin.

And the time I was holding my second born while checking the pilot light on the water heater, and his arm touched the scalding hot pipe of the nearby furnace, which gave him a small burn about the size of a staple. And a thousand other moments when I learned something I hadn't known before. While these moments were pretty brutal for me (and likely for my sons as well), they were also somewhat typical new-parent moments. Wisdom is born from making mistakes and learning from them. You can't know what you didn't know before you knew it. Parenting involves a lot of trial and error. You learn as you go, and learning involves messing up.

Practice Self-Forgiveness

Possibly the most important skills to develop as a new parent are self-compassion and self-forgiveness. These are as necessary as cutting yourself some slack and developing humility. It takes a huge amount of strength to admit to and *forgive* yourself for making mistakes. Maybe mistakes don't even exist since each one teaches you something new.

When my kids were about four and two years old, I was trying to get them dressed on a particularly challenging morning. They were both in horrible moods—crying and complaining—while I was tee-tering on the edge of losing it. At one point, I stopped, looked at them both, and firmly stated, "Mommy needs a time-out." I got up and left the room to take a much-needed break . . . *but they followed me!* As they got close, I started to run. There I was running down the hall-way with two screaming toddlers following after me. I'm sure we were quite the sight! I ran into my bathroom and into my closet, closing the door behind me as best I could with all the bathrobes and jackets hanging in the way, which prevented the door from actually shutting. I sat on the floor with my back to the door, stuck my fingers in my ears, and sang "la la la la la" out loud while my two boys banged on the door, wailing to be let in!

I desperately needed a break, and this was the only way I could think of in the moment to get one. My kids were safe and the sixty seconds or so that I took while sitting on the floor of my closet was necessary for my well-being. At first, when I told my husband about my closet time-out, I thought of it as a bad parenting moment, but soon I was able to not only forgive myself for being human and needing a break but to see the hilarity of the situation! When you have your version of the closet time-out, forgive yourself for being human and congratulate yourself on remembering to take breaks.

Stay in the Moment

There is a tendency to flash forward and ask yourself questions like, "If I can't figure out how to get my baby to eat, how will I ever be able to teach them math?" Let yourself learn to roll over before expecting yourself to run. Your skills as a parent will grow over time and will develop alongside your baby. You don't have to know *now* how to help your child do difficult math, go on their first date, handle a bully, go off to college, or any other parenting milestone that comes much further down the parenting path. You only have to do today or even this moment. Address the challenges in an appropriate time frame. If for you that means looking ahead to the next likely developmental milestone, go for it, but you don't need to fret over how your child will adjust to being away from you at kindergarten when they aren't yet eating solid food. Keep your perspective and stay in this moment, right now.

Expand Your Expectations

Before you have a child, it's pretty easy to believe parenting isn't that hard. There's a meme going around social media that says, "Parenting was so much easier when I was raising my nonexistent children hypothetically." Parenting is hard, and many people only learn just *how* hard it is *after* they have kids themselves. Before I had kids, I never believed I would ever let my kid wail if I had any choice to do otherwise. But then I found myself taking a much-needed shower while my son screamed his heart out lying on a towel on the bathroom floor just outside the shower. Often expectations around what you should be able to tolerate are just too damn high!

Drop the idea that you will or even *should* enjoy every moment. Parents of older kids often give the same well-meaning advice to new parents: "Enjoy every minute as they grow up fast." My kids are now both nearly launched. They are mature and connecting adults that I love dearly and enjoy spending time with. But did I enjoy every minute? Hell no! That shit's pure fantasy!

I remember when my kids were little. Parenting was a challenging, bring-me-to-my-knees slog for years on end, peppered with joyful moments and memorable celebrations. Early parenting required the endurance and tenacity of a triathlete or Himalayan trekker. There were many moments of joy, lots of struggles, and millions of unremarkable moments long forgotten with time.

Parents with adult or nearly adult children often romanticize the days of infancy, remembering the cute cheeks, the giggles, and the numerous "firsts," but at the same time, they forget the sleepless nights, breastfeeding struggles, loneliness, identity crises, productivity challenges, and the feeling that it will never, ever, end.

The advice to "enjoy every minute as they grow up fast" comes from the altitude of arriving at the top of the parenting mountain and looking back over the journey as one who has survived. When you're just starting the parenting trek, struggling to take the first steps and surviving the first long months of the journey, being told to enjoy every minute can invalidate the lived experience and cause new parents to wonder how they're doing it wrong. They feel they must be doing it wrong, they have to be, or else how could someone who has already completed this mountainous climb tell them to "enjoy" what can feel like hell?

As with childbirth, there is no single golden ticket that guarantees a smooth parenting journey. Many things help, such as gaining experience and developing new skills, having supportive people around, and a bit of luck that your child's disposition and needs match well with what you are able to offer them. Expand your expectations about parenthood. As you did in preparation for childbirth, strategize not just how to relax when the waters are calm and the sky blue, but also imagine what might help you navigate the rapids when the river of parenting becomes demanding and tough.

Soften Your Attachments

As you settle into parenting, certain activities become habits, accidental successes become required daily elements, and attachment to helpful tricks and tools gets set in concrete. Attachment is a sly and insidious shadow in parenthood, hooking us when our guard is down and when we are especially vulnerable. While we need hope, attachment to a particular outcome breeds misery. As soon as something becomes easier—your baby sleeps for a longer stretch, a feeding goes well, you make a successful trip to the grocery store, and so on—the common response is to become attached to it happening the same way again or from then on. Similarly, when a day or night is particularly hard, we attach to it *not* happening that way again. Attachment to a particular future creates suffering.

Change is constant, especially in the first year of a child's life. Developmental milestones exist around every corner bringing shifting behavior, fluctuating moods, and new concerns. Babies change. The good news is that whatever the difficulty, it likely won't last forever. The bad news is that the easy parts are likely to go through changes too. When I meet with new parents around six weeks after their baby is born, it's common for some parents to express their surprise at how much their baby sleeps. If I meet with those same parents when their baby is three to four months old and going through a big developmental change, they will likely tell me something very different about their child's sleep habits. Hold all your expectations and attachments lightly.

As in childbirth, parenting constantly challenges our notions of control and power. Parenting is a relationship between at least two people; as such, it is unpredictable and often unruly. Preferences on all sides abound. Children are not computers into which you can insert a line of code to produce a particular predictable behavior. Parenting is a practice in nonattachment.

When my kids were babies, my husband and I would sing particular lullabies to them at bedtime. The song we sang every night for over two years was one I learned while trekking in the Himalayas in my early twenties. I loved it and was emotionally attached to it. At some point in my older son's second year, we added additional songs to our nighttime routine including "Baa, Baa, Black Sheep." The day came when our son no longer wanted to hear the song we loved and had come to associate with sweet bedtimes. At that point, all we ever got to sing was "Baa, Baa, Black Sheep"—10,000 times! Maybe I was being overly sentimental, but it was still a practice in letting go of attachments.

Ask for and Accept Help

Asking for help falls under the heading of parenting as a profound personal practice because for many modern people, asking for help is hard to do. In a society that bestows names like "Superman" and "Goddess" to parents who can "do it all," asking for help is often unconsciously engrained as a sign of weakness. Nothing could be further from the truth. Parenting truly takes a whole group of people, a village, as the saying goes, as well as reduced expectations. The values of an Apollonian society tend to keep expectations high and judgment about needing help loaded. Modern industrialized culture lives removed from extended family and agricultural life where parents worked near or around the home. Add to that the need and/or desire for both parents to have a career, and you begin to get a picture of the stress modern parents feel raising kids. The work of parenting now falls more and more on people who *already* have limited time and resources within a culture whose message is not only that you can do it all, but that you should smile while doing so.

Instead, modern parents need to practice asking for and accepting help from others. When someone offers to help you with your groceries, practice accepting the help. If friends or family come over for dinner, ask them to help with dishes. You do not have to do it all on your own. The proverbial village rarely just shows up. We have to ask it to come to our aid.

Nurture a Kind Inner Voice

In the end, when you've tried what you can try, done what you can do, and you still feel the intensity of parenting washing over you, practice speaking kindly to yourself. Imagine that you are a little child who is completely dependent on you for love and attention. Speak to yourself the way you would a scared child or a wounded animal. Hold yourself gently with words of tenderness. Develop a kind inner voice. It is one of the only voices that quiets the inner judge and critic.

"I'd like to encourage us all to lighten up, to practice with a lot of gentleness. This is not the drill sergeant saying, 'Lighten up or else.' I have found that if we can possibly use anything we hear against ourselves, we usually do." PEMA CHÖDRÖN[5]

When I use this inner voice, it speaks to me as if someone else were speaking the words. This is one of the tricks I use to bypass the "woe is me" voice that can whine inside my own mind! Try sentences like these in a tender and loving inner tone of voice:

- You're trying so hard.

- You wish it were easier.

- This is so much harder than you thought it would be.

- You're doing the best you can.

- It's okay to wish it were different.

- You wish you knew then what you know now.

- This matters so much to you, and it's still hard.

- You are enough, even when you don't feel like it.

- You are still loveable.

Write some of your own. What helps you remember the full truth of who you are even when you're struggling? If the wisest, kindest, most nurturing person were to say loving and helpful words to you during difficult moments, what would they say? Practice developing this inner voice and use it frequently.

Sometimes, we judge ourselves then judge ourselves for judging ourselves, and so on. Even if it's well down a path of self-criticism, try unhooking the chain of self-judgment. Wherever it's possible to do so, unhook the criticism, and then add tenderness to the voice that judged you to begin with. There's no point in judging the inner critic too—even that part of us deserves to be held with tenderness.

One Step at a Time

Remember that parenting skills don't develop overnight, nor do abilities to traverse personally challenging realms of parenthood. Both develop and grow moment by moment. When embraced as a growth-based journey, it's easier to remember there are good days and bad days, days when you feel connected to all that is good, and days where you feel dragged through the muck. These are normal fluctuations on any profound personal path. Trust that each day, and through each new experience, you are growing. And that matters—a lot.

Couples Who
Are Parents

Too little is discussed regarding how having a baby will impact your relationship. This chapter addresses that topic head on. If you are not in a romantic relationship, you may still find the practices and guidance in this chapter helpful.

THE TRUTH ABOUT BRINGING A BABY INTO YOUR RELATIONSHIP

Becoming parents changes your relationship and not always for the better. Let's not sugar coat this. Many books address how amazing it is to see your partner hold your child or the profound experience of witnessing the unfolding skill of their parenting. Social media, parenting and pregnancy magazines, and even Hollywood are filled with images of beautifully coiffed couples gazing lovingly at their precious bundle of joy while oozing love between them.

Yes . . . profound, love-filled moments unfurl on the wind of new parenthood, and those moments can help parents stay connected to one another. However, the myth that having a baby will definitely make your relationship *better* is simply not supported by the research.

Many couples report a decline in relationship satisfaction after the birth of a baby (between 43 and 83 percent depending on the study), for some the satisfaction remained relatively stable (about 39 percent), and a few, about 18 percent, experienced an increase in their satisfaction after the birth of a baby.[1] And if you think these statistics don't apply to you because you and your partner have chosen not to get married (or are in an area that restricts your ability to do so) or have adopted rather than birthed your baby, think again. The research shows that there is no difference in satisfaction between married and unmarried couples.[2] Having children challenges relationships across family structures and circumstances.

I share these statistics not to scare you or cloud your excitement heading into parenthood, but rather to pop the bubble of innocent beliefs in order to motivate you to do the necessary work for the benefit of your relationship. Let's explore some ways to prepare and strengthen your relationship so it weathers the challenges resiliently.

Expanding Your Expectations

Part of the process of preparation is expanding your expectations around those images of family-centric, bliss-filled love fests! Not that those moments won't happen. They most likely will. But unlike life *before* baby, in life after baby, the dominant energy of the relationship shifts from lovers to co-parents, and the focus shifts from the couple to the family. Family-centric connection fulfills many of our needs for intimacy, but it is important to remember that the relationship, as a separate and unique entity, has needs beyond those of the family.

Before my husband, Brent, and I got married, we focused on making our relationship strong enough to handle whatever came our way. We were young, in love, and dedicated to our daily predawn yoga practice. From early on, we used our relationship as a place for growth and personal practice. Our relationship blossomed next to each other on yoga mats, so the idea of relationship *as practice* made sense to us. We consciously worked at our relationship. Until that point in my life, I believed, as so many of us do—consciously or unconsciously—that if you just find the "right person" it will all be easy.

Let me just clear that fairy tale up right here: It's simply bullshit! Relationships, even without the added stresses of parenthood, require effort and care, and during early parenthood, relationships face extra challenges.

Exhaustion and Sleep Deprivation

Acknowledge and expect to be tired in early parenthood. When we are tired, we rarely share our best selves with those around us, especially those with whom we are comfortable. Raw edges and sharp tongues tend to accompany the dark circles under the eyes. When we are exhausted, we also tend to be emotionally tender. As such, things that might not upset us when we are fully rested can cut to the core. It can be helpful to know and remember this truth. If your partner is more emotional, biting, or edgy during the first year, lack of sleep may be the cause. Try seeing beneath the rough edges to the exposed tender place from where the nasty behavior likely arises. Rather than fighting with a partner who is being unkind, it is often more helpful to express concern, curiosity, and tenderness.

Emotional Instability

Beyond sleep deprivation are the impacts of changing hormones, new experiences, and added stress, all of which add to emotional instability. Like labor, postpartum is a time of changing and shifting moods. Remember the river metaphor in chapter 7? After giving birth, new parents are still in the river, with its variability, instability, and changing emotions. Just like they needed in labor, after birth birthing parents need strong, understanding, and supportive banks that remind them that this too is okay, and that they are loved through the shifting waters of the postpartum period.

The shifting emotional landscape is particularly common in the first week after the baby is born. According to postpartum expert Dr. Aviva Romm, "the postpartum hormone drop is considered the single largest sudden hormone change in the shortest amount of time for any human being, at any point of their life cycle."[3] This drop tends to occur around the time the breast milk comes in. The massive drop in estrogen and progesterone tends to make the birthing parent highly sensitive, profoundly tender, and often weepy—an experience known as the "baby blues." One minute they may be filled with love for the new baby and the next a puddle of tears. The baby blues usually subside within a week or so as the body adjusts to the hormonal shifts. The baby blues is not the same thing as postpartum depression.

Sometimes, parents need more than the support a partner or other loved one can provide. Postpartum depression, anxiety, post-traumatic stress, obsessive-compulsive disorder, and psychosis are all experiences that can happen to either partner from when the baby is born through the first year of the baby's life. These conditions are often either lumped together as postpartum mood disorders or erroneously as postpartum depression, since it is the most broadly known of the bunch. Any of these conditions can be hard on your relationship and should be treated with care, attention, and professional help. Don't try to go it alone. If you notice signs in yourself or your partner that may include anxiety, anger, sleeping difficulty (even when you have the chance), or profound sadness, get help. Postpartum mood disorders are common and very often treatable. Keep in mind that reliable, practical, and emotional support during the postpartum period can help reduce the incidence of postpartum mood disorders in the first place.

Demands on Your Time

Also challenging to your relationship are the increased demands on your time and energy. Not only do you still have many of the obligations you had before having a baby, such as work, household chores, personal care, and sleep, but now you also have to take care of a completely dependent infant. Bringing a baby into your family adds complexity and volume to everything—there is now more laundry, a greater necessity for good hygiene and nutrition, and fewer hours of sleep. The extra time needed to care for a new baby has to come from somewhere and often comes from the time you might otherwise have spent with your partner. Having a baby means having to consciously remember to tend to your relationship.

TENDING THE RELATIONSHIP GARDEN

Relationships take work, effort, commitment, flexibility, resilience, and stamina. They thrive on love, acceptance, humor, openness, and play. Never is this truer than in the months and years following the birth of a child. Relationships, like a garden, need tilling, tending, pruning, fertilizing, moisture, and sunshine.

One of the concepts that Brent and I learned early in our relationship was the idea of the relationship as its own entity.[4] There's Brent. There's me. And there's our relationship, which is its own thing, separate from the wants and needs of either of the individuals who make it up. I have my needs and preferences, Brent has his, and our relationship has its own as well.

When things are easy, all of our desires line up and flow together. Those moments are blissful. Struggle comes when the two parties have conflicting needs and wishes. When this happens, the needs of the relationship are often sidelined, while the focus is placed on *personal* wants. Surprisingly, what usually helps a couple through the conflict is turning toward the relationship and inquiring about what the relationship needs, separate from individual desires. For us, conflict was far easier to navigate when we paused in building our personal side of the argument and opened to the possibility that there was another truth, another need being voiced by the relationship that was separate but often entangled with the unmet needs being expressed by each of our personal sides.

What's tougher to notice, and therefore covertly dangerous, is when the two individuals' needs are being met, but the relationship is ignored. One of the ways this showed up for us was in how we spent our evenings after our baby was asleep. I was perfectly happy to spend some time alone focusing on my professional or personal passions. I'm someone who loves time alone and needs it for my emotional well-being, and nights felt like my only chance to nourish my need for solitude. When we were new parents, Brent was also starting a business and growing his career. For him, the work never seemed to end, and there was always something he could do for work after our baby was asleep. We were each happy to tend to these other needs independently. We're both hard workers and can easily get lost in the desire to get more done. Our needs were not in conflict, but the relationship—the space between us—was being ignored. Too many nights of doing our own thing often led to distance in the relationship. This is true for us to this day. We each have thriving careers, a robust family life, and the desire to get a lot done, but we still have to remember to create time for our relationship.

It takes intention and attention to support an intimate relationship through the testing ground of new parenthood, but *there is good news*: by turning toward your relationship rather than away from it, you can actually come through those early years closer and stronger as a couple than ever before. I know it's possible, because we did it. Here are some additional ways to support your relationship; some we used through early parenthood, and others we learned along the way.

Relationship Rituals

Relationship experts John and Julie Gottman say that to help relationships thrive they need "small things often."[5] While I've only recently become familiar with the Gottmans' work, this concept is one Brent and I have used throughout our relationship. I think of these acts as relationship rituals—small things done frequently to support the relationship. These can be as simple as a hug, words of appreciation, and/or sharing aspects of childcare and the workload around your home. Small frequent acts make a far bigger overall difference than grand gestures that rarely happen.

Try incorporating rituals into your relationship that support connection in a nonsexual way. There are several ways to do this. Here are a few I have used personally or cocreated with couples I've worked with.

Thresholds

As new parents, coming back together after being apart is a particularly good time to establish a relationship-supporting ritual. If one parent has been home most of the day alone with the baby while the other parent has been working, each of you has expectations and needs upon coming back together. Unexpressed and unmet expectations can lead to resentment. Discuss what you each need when you first come together after time apart.

One couple I worked with kept running into problems after work. The mother, who was home with their child all day, was desperate for her husband to take the baby the second he walked in the door. The husband had a highly physical and emotionally taxing job and desperately needed a shower to both clean himself off and to have five minutes alone to process his day before he could really be available to his family. Once they discussed this and began to understand what each of them needed, they developed some rituals that supported their connection and relationship. What worked for them was to have the husband come home and go directly to the shower. He was not to get sidetracked by the mail or phone messages or even his wife and child. Once he had showered, they agreed that he would come directly out and take the baby for thirty minutes so that the mom could have time completely to herself. After the thirty minutes, they would come together and say hello, connect, hug, and acknowledge each other as partners, not just as co-parents and roommates.

Another couple I worked with made a ritual of crossing the threshold of their home, and as soon as they saw each other after being apart for a time, the very first thing they would do is greet one another as lovers. They would hug and kiss, look into each other's eyes, and have a moment of remembering who they were to each other beyond their roles as parents. Only after they greeted each other would the one who had been away greet their child. This turned the center of their relationship from co-parents to lovers even though they hadn't yet resumed a sexual relationship after birth. They noticed a profound change in their positive feelings for one another after only a few days of this practice.

That couple's practice was very similar to what Brent and I incorporated as well. It wasn't always easy. There were days when Brent would come home ready to "connect" as he crossed the threshold, and I would be agitated by whatever was happening in the moment, be it a pot of boiling water for pasta, an upset baby, an email demanding my attention, or my own exhaustion. Pausing and softening to connect almost always helped interrupt any negative spin I might be in the midst of. Connecting also reminded me that I wasn't alone in the challenges of parenthood. That made a difference in my ability to ask for and receive help.

Mealtimes

Mealtimes are another great place to establish rituals that support your relationship and will likely develop into rituals that support your family as time passes and children grow. Make agreements about cell phone use at mealtimes—maybe have phone-free dinners every night or just on Fridays. You get to decide together. Or try making one meal a week a time when you talk very specifically about what's happening in your individual lives. During this meal each of you gets to share from the heart about your work, life, joys, and challenges, while the other parent listens. Especially for women, intimacy often starts by talking *and* feeling heard.

Eye Gazing

One practice that my husband and I use is eye gazing. While it can feel strange at first, it is a powerful practice of connection. Try it for three minutes and see what happens.

Here's how you do it:

Sit facing your partner close enough that you can comfortably look into each other's eyes. Hold hands or let your knees touch. Settle into a relaxed gaze, resting your focus on your partner's left eye. Let your breath slow and just be with your partner. That's it. Setting a timer can help. I recommend starting with three to five minutes and building up to ten or even fifteen minutes. Close the eye-gazing session ritually by blowing out a candle, bowing to one another, or with words of appreciation.

Hugs and Embraces

Many couples find it helpful to move toward more intimate physical contact slowly. Try hugging, embracing, or snuggling as a way to connect physically, but without sexual contact. Of course, both partners have to agree to this practice. Try adding hugs into your day and a cuddle while watching a show together or as you fall asleep. Finding ways to connect physically is important for many relationships. That connection does not have to be intercourse. Expand beyond limiting ideas of genital contact as the only mode for loving physical contact and connection.

Massage

Similar to hugs and cuddling, massage can be a great way to slowly find your way back to one another physically. Trade off giving each other physical pleasure without any focus on genital sex. Give a hand or foot rub—five minutes for each hand or foot—or give your partner a ten-minute shoulder or back rub just before bed, then switch giver and receiver the next night. Break connection into smaller, easy-to-accomplish pieces rather than giant unrealistic tasks that require a lot of effort.

Sensual Touch

Adding sexual connection back into your relationship after having a baby can be challenging for some new parents. Try starting by adding sensual touch *without* sexual intentions. Make your touch, caress, and/or conversation about connecting more intimately, *not* about sex specifically. If one partner has imbued sex with acceptance, love, and need, or feels starved for physical contact post-baby, you'll likely need to have an explicit understanding and mutual agreement *before you start* that this practice is not to progress to sex. This agreement helps remove any uncertainty about how this session will end. Uncertainty can make sensual touch uncomfortable for someone who wants to connect but doesn't feel ready for sex. Setting a timer for a specific amount of time and taking turns giving and receiving can be helpful.

Be Creative

What other relationship rituals can you incorporate into your relationship post-baby? Get creative. If you are used to walking around the block with your dog before dinner, maybe you can continue that with baby in a stroller or carrier. Perhaps you like to go to the movies every Friday. Can you instead find a few movies you can stream and watch at home together? Maybe you already have a relationship ritual that feeds your intimacy and connection. If so, keep it going and come up with creative ways of modifying it to work for both of you after your baby arrives. Whether it's maintaining a relationship ritual or starting a new one, make a realistic commitment to your relationship now that you can continue long into parenthood.

Guardian of the Relationship

It is far too easy after having a baby to forget to turn attention toward your relationship as a couple. For my husband and me, after having one baby and then another, going out became more difficult for a variety of reasons—we had to line up childcare and have enough physical and emotional energy to make it worthwhile, and we had to let go of micromanaging how our babies were cared for while we were out. I struggled with the idea of anyone else being able to care for our baby and had zero extra energy to expend on figuring out childcare! Our relationship needed time and focused attention. Brent was able to see that better than I could as I was caught in the haze of early motherhood. He took it on himself to make sure we got out together, without our kids.

We described his role in this as "guardian of the relationship." He watched out for the well-being of our relationship in those early days, making sure it got the attention it needed. This was so helpful to me. Brent would carefully consider who would work best for childcare, often asking grandmothers for help. He would check in with me, but did all the heavy lifting when it came to planning. The first few dates he planned were simple and short. We built our ability to take time away from our babies and make time for our relationship slowly and deliberately.

Going out is not required to give focused time and attention to your relationship. At-home dates can be just as wonderful if held with conscious boundaries and intentions for what the time is to be used for. Take-out meals eaten on a picnic blanket in front of a fire or by candlelight can be as wonderful if not even better than a meal out in a restaurant. Don't let a lack of good childcare or financial resources keep you from putting deliberate attention on your relationship. Set time aside to turn toward one another.

Relationship Communication Practices

Be aware that at first it is common for conversation on "dates" to circle around *the baby*. This is both typical and okay. Yes, it is important to remember yourselves beyond the baby, but it is also important to remember that the baby is a huge part of your lives. What's worse is that if you attempt to avoid talking about the baby, you might inadvertently mute the voice and experience of the primary caregiver whose day-to-day existence is highly wrapped up with the topic of the baby. If you notice the tendency to focus only on the baby, try opening the conversation to the parent's personal experience of parenting rather than the baby as the topic itself. Here are a few suggestions for enhancing your shared communication.

Open-Ended Questions

Use daily conversations as well as dates to check in with each other's lives. One of the key stressors on relationships after a baby is born is a loss of understanding and involvement in each other's lives, which in turn, can lead to distance, misunderstanding, and resentment. Relationships benefit from mutual sharing about your independent lives. Open-ended questions are great for provoking discussions of this sort. Try asking questions like the following with curiosity and without believing you already know the likely answer:

- Can you describe how you spend your time when we're not together?

- What's the best part of how you spend your time?

- What's the hardest part of how you spend your time?

- What was new or different for you this week?

- What current challenges are you working through and how are you facing those challenges?

There are many others, but I think you get the idea. Make up your own and get curious. Assuming you know what happens in your partner's daily life can be dangerous. Genuine curiosity is powerful and helpful in creating intimacy and building strong relationships.

Staying Current

One of the things that got us into trouble early in our relationship was holding on to bad feelings. If I got mad at Brent and shared my upset with him, I would often hold on to my story of what happened long after it had dissipated. Even after I'd cleared the upset with him, I would find myself still hanging on to my feelings about it rather than allowing myself to be in the new emotion that had replaced it. The inverse was also true. I would sometimes not let myself be fully angry or upset about something that my rational brain brushed off as insignificant. Both of these habits were breeding grounds for resentment and bad feelings.

A teacher we worked with taught us about being fully in the experience while it's happening—when angry, be angry—when the anger passes, let it go. I started practicing being truer to my emotions in the moment, as they were, without attachment to needing them to be different. Doing so meant I had to pay closer attention to exactly what I was feeling in any given moment. In this way, I was practicing being the water of the river again . . . changing and flowing with the emotion of the moment. By unhooking from the story and instead staying with the feelings, I could move toward healing the relationship rupture more quickly. Conversely, it also helped me share my feelings with Brent when they were small rather than letting them fester and grow into ugly, unruly monsters of resentment. This would have been a good practice for Brent too, but he didn't need it as much as I did. He was already better at rolling with what he felt when he felt it.

Relationship Repair

Staying current also allows for the practice of repair to take root. Probably one of the most important practices within our relationship is the practice of conscious relationship repair.

I don't know about you, but when I'm fired up, I tend to tighten my body, hold my breath, and either talk rapidly or clam up. Addressing heated issues with Brent when either of us is in this state is rarely a good idea. When we have the awareness to do so, usually all we need to unhook from the intensity is to insert a pause, take a breath, and intentionally soften our bodies.

If you notice that something you said or did inspired a negative response from your partner, ask for a do-over. Brent and I will often say, "Let me try that again." Alternatively, when one of us has heard something that didn't sit well, we try and share what we heard back to our partner to make sure we are actually hearing the message they intended. Miscommunication can happen easily in relationship, but that doesn't mean we should hold fast to what they said or did without the opportunity for repair.

Necessary for relationship repair is the willingness to admit mistakes and say, "I'm sorry." Offering and receiving forgiveness helps heal tears in the fabric of relationships. Forgiving and moving on are important for the longevity of relationships. As the saying goes, "Shit happens, and life goes on." It could be said that shit happens, and relationships need to repair to go on and thrive. Repair and forgiveness are relationship practices. The more you integrate them into your interactions, the stronger the skills will become.

Talking Circle

Before we were married, Brent and I had the good fortune to be introduced to a special and ritualized communication practice that we have used throughout our relationship as a couple and have brought into our family life as well. It has been key to the success of our marriage and our family communication, including navigating difficult conflicts.

Council, as it was called when Brent and I learned it from teachers at the Ojai Foundation, is a nonhierarchical practice of sitting in circle with the intention of listening deeply and speaking from the heart.[6] It calls to mind the image from chapter 1 of ancient people sitting together around a fire with respect and attentiveness.

According to Lewis Mehl-Medrona and Barbara Mainguy, today talking circles are used to facilitate nonhierarchical, egalitarian, and nonreactionary conversations in schools, families, communities, political groups, health-care settings, and therapeutic programs. And even though talking circles are now utilized in many different communities and settings, the roots of this practice are found in traditional practices of Native Americans in the United States and the First Nations people of Canada. Mehl-Medrona and Mainguy say that "traditionally, many Native American communities have used the talking circle as a way of bringing people of all ages together for the purposes of teaching, listening, and learning . . . This method of education instilled respect for another's viewpoint and encouraged members to be open to other viewpoints by listening with their hearts while another individual speaks."[7] Even with its widespread use, its roots must be acknowledged and respected. I am forever grateful that I was instructed in this practice as it has profoundly impacted my life. I share it with you below, with deepest respect and gratitude to its creators.[8]

Try This

Practicing Council

The ritual of this practice is part of what makes it profoundly powerful and effective. Gather together a candle, something to light it with, and an item you can use as a talking piece, which is something that denotes whose turn it is to speak. Select an item that holds some amount of significance to both of you, such as an adorned stick, a special rock, or some other sacred item. Select a comfortable place to sit that is different from where you would normally sit with your partner to chat, have a meal, or watch TV. My family sits on floor chairs in the middle of our living room, which is something that we only do for council. Setting up the sacred space is critical. Doing so triggers you into a different mode right from the beginning. Your mind notices the difference, wakes up, and brings to attention your wisest self.

Sit across from your partner or, if you are practicing with others such as your children or extended family, sit in a circle. Place the candle at the center and put the item you've selected to designate the speaker next to the candle. Take a few moments to settle into your seat and into the moment. Notice your breath. Create a noticeable pause in the activity of both your body and mind. When you have both settled, light the candle. Once the candle is lit, certain rules are observed: only the person with the talking piece may speak, no one can interrupt, and no one can leave the circle until the session is finished. End times can either be agreed upon beforehand or sessions can be open-ended, coming to a conclusion when both parties feel the session is done.

Beyond the rules, there are intentions to hold within the practice. Make it your intention to listen deeply, to speak from your heart, to stay in the present moment, and to be as brief as possible—only holding the talking piece long enough to express what is needed in the moment.[9] Staying in the present moment is perhaps the hardest part of council, as it means you don't plan how you're going to respond to what you hear while listening. You get to respond in the moment when you have the talking piece. When you come to the end, either after a pre-agreed upon amount of time or when the session comes to a natural stopping point, blow out the candle. Brent and I then like to take a moment to breathe together, look in each other's eyes, or hug.

I recommend couples new to this council ritual make a commitment to practice regularly: once a week, once every two weeks, or once a month are all reasonable commitments for practice. You will know what will work for your lifestyle as well as support your relationship in the way it needs. Initially, Brent and I sat in circle together regularly whether or not we felt we needed it. Making it a scheduled regular practice helped establish council as foundational to our relationship. Today, we don't have this practice marked on our calendars, but it has been such a core part of our relationship for a couple of decades that we trust we will call on it whenever it is needed.

In addition to scheduled times, either partner can call a circle anytime they feel one is needed or desired. This doesn't mean that dropping into a communication circle must happen in that very moment, but it does mean scheduling one as soon as it can be arranged. Sometimes, sitting in circle resolves whatever it is that brings you to the chairs. Other times, it opens the topic but does not bring any resolution. The Gottmans state that 69 percent of relationship problems are recurrent and are not resolvable.[10] The topics that come up are often ones that repeat, and finding ways to safely contain and discuss "hot button" issues is what's really beneficial about this practice.

Further down the path of parenting, you might find this practice to be helpful with your children. Sitting together as equals, even when our kids were little, was a powerful family practice for us. Our kids knew that if they had something scary to share or wanted to be sure they were deeply heard, they could call us all to circle. Some of our family communication circles were deep and others verged on hilarious. Many are emblazoned in my memory profoundly.

Relationship Primacy

I already addressed extended family in chapter 11, but navigating relationships with extended family is one of the most common topics brought up by couples when they come to me for guidance before and after the birth of a baby. Dealing with in-laws can be an added stress on the relationship between new parents. This is especially true when grandparents have opinions that differ from those of the parents and attempt to get their child to agree with them.

Let me give you an example. When a couple I know had a new baby, the parents decided to sleep train when their baby was a few months old. The father's mother thought this was a bad idea and worked to convince her son that sleep training was detrimental. This put the new dad in a very tricky situation where his mother and his wife were at odds with one another, and he was stuck between two people he loved.

I believe it is important for couples to center their relationship and make it primary. That means, you make decisions together as a couple and decide *together* who to ask for parenting guidance. Turning toward the relationship helps develop a stronger partnership between parents in the co-parenting process. Make supporting your partner a higher priority than pleasing your parents or other well-meaning advice givers. Your relationship will benefit from actions that place your partner and your relationship closer to the center of importance.

Addressing Parenting Differences

Another critical area of discussion for couples is about differences in parenting styles. So important is this topic that when my husband and I lead relationship workshops for new parents, this is one of the four main modules we address. Many of the relationship challenges new parents bring to work on in private sessions with me have something to do with differences in parenting styles. Conflicts over how to raise children are common, but they don't need to be catastrophic. Utilizing many of the tools shared in this chapter will help you navigate disagreements and challenges in this arena. In addition to what I've already shared, here are a few other suggestions for supporting your family through parenting style differences.

Identify Shared Parenting Values

Many parents complain that they aren't on the same page as their partner in regard to childrearing practices. I believe being on the same page is completely overrated. You don't have to be on the same page; however being in the same chapter or at least the same book is very helpful. To that end, I recommend reading a parenting book or two together. If reading together is unlikely to happen, try taking a baby-care class together, listening to a podcast together or, if nothing else, talk about what is important to each of you in raising your children. Work to come up with a few key elements that resonate for both of you. These can include conversations around childcare possibilities, what to do when your baby is upset or crying, sleeping arrangements, what types of toys, books, and/or media you want your child to be exposed to and at what age, and also discipline, food, education, religion, and holidays. Starting with these topics can help you figure out some of your shared values around parenting and building a family.

Making decisions as a couple involves a lot of compromise. Learning when to lead and when to listen is part of the co-parenting journey. As you become more familiar with what matters to you and your partner, you each grow in your understanding of the other. Use this growing understanding to soften judgment and to help navigate co-parenting disagreements.

Staying Open

What happens when you aren't in alignment with your partner? First, ask yourself if the topic of disagreement is important. Remember that there are two parents. As simple and obvious as this might seem, it is the best advice I can give you. Each of us has our own way of doing the same thing. The way my husband held our boys when they were babies was *not* the same way I did. But does that mean his way was wrong because it wasn't *my* way? No. His way was his, and my way was mine. Our boys were safe in the arms of either of us and that was what really mattered. That doesn't mean there weren't times I told (or wanted to tell) my husband to change the way he held our sons. But just because I was the one who spent the majority of my time with our children didn't mean I got to trump all of his parenting choices or got to be the expert from whom all instruction flowed.

Part of my personal practice as a co-parent came in returning over and over again to the awareness that my way was not the *only* right way. It was my way, and Brent's way was his way, and neither way was better than the other. So long as our children were safe, emotionally and physically, we could agree to disagree on smaller issues.

Where it got particularly dicey were the moments when our parenting styles clashed specifically because we had different definitions and comfort levels around what it meant to be safe. This area of conflict continues to challenge us to this day now that our children are driving cars and traveling to far-off places in the world . . . issues no more real than the early challenges around holding baby's head and proper bath time safety. In these areas, Brent and I have agreed to hear each other's concerns and practice staying open to the possibility that the other may have a valid point. That's it. Practice staying open.

Both of us know that I am the more safety-conscious parent. And we both also acknowledge that my anxiety regarding safety is in part fueled by family tragedy that tends to cause me to be overly, and sometimes unnecessarily, alarmed. That same fuel also causes me to see things that are potentially dangerous that Brent does not. There have been times when I have shared my concern with Brent about a safety issue, and he has changed his mind and agreed with me. At other times, he has asked me to respect his take on the situation, and I have lessened my standards, trusting that he's got it. This dance of respect and openness has gotten us through many potential conflicts.

Sex

At some point as you exit the postpartum labyrinth, the conversation about and/or the desire for sex arises. This can be a challenging point in the labyrinth for many parents. If a baby has come out of your vagina, it can be daunting to imagine anything going back in there! If your baby was born surgically, the healing journey may be longer than anticipated and feeling extra vulnerable is common. Additionally, many breastfeeding parents feel touched out and even the idea of being touched by their intimate partner is more than they can handle. For others, giving birth and nursing a baby can feel highly sensual and the desire for erotic contact is heightened by the experience. There isn't one way that sexual desire, or lack thereof, presents itself during postpartum.

Similarly, some partners feel exhausted by the experience of early parenthood and can't imagine having enough energy to be sexually intimate. Others may be impacted by witnessing birth and have a difficult time envisioning the vagina as a sexual organ after having witnessed its reproductive power. Still others may be so blown away by the intensity of birth that their awe impacts their sexual desire. And many partners are eager to resume sexual intimacy far sooner than the birthing parent feels ready.

The key thing to remember about sexual intimacy is that it is a type of connection but by no means the *only* one. Both parents need to be ready to reengage in sexual intimacy, and it cannot nor should be forced on either partner. Building connection and closeness is key to a healthy relationship postpartum. Be sure to practice open communication around what is pleasing and what is not. Clear, open, and honest communication is vital for the safe and pleasurable return to sexual intimacy after baby.

Take time and incorporate exercises and practices to help bring you back to a sexually fulfilling relationship as a couple (those listed earlier are a great place to start). It is also helpful to expand beyond genital-to-genital intercourse. Often it is easier to begin with sensual touch, hand to genital stimulation, or oral sex before going back to penetrative intercourse. After having a baby is a great time to expand your sexual focus to include activities and practices beyond penetrative sex.

In addition to what I've already shared for you as a couple, there are individual practices that can help the union with your partner feel more natural and open when you choose to come together sexually, but are practiced alone. We will address connecting with your individual sexual self in the next chapter.

RELATIONSHIP AS SPIRITUAL PRACTICE

I view parenting as a profound spiritual practice. Parenting with another person doubles that practice. Here's what I can tell you from the vantage point of nearing the end of the intensive parenting years . . . when the kids have flown off into the future of their creation, your partner just might still be there with you and that's a pretty amazing thing. For me, parenting has actually been a more easeful spiritual practice. I took to it pretty quickly and found it somewhat easy to laugh at my foibles. But relationship tests my mettle, my flexibility, my commitment to growth, and my ideas about who I am.

Brent is my partner. We have worked together to raise two children, built careers and a home, and loved, laughed, fought, and healed together through many challenges. He's uniquely gifted at driving me a bit crazy. But that's relationship for you. Your partner is likely your personal crazy-maker!

I wish for you the ability to see the challenges that will arise in your relationship as opportunities to grow, deepen, and expand. My mom calls her marriage a "workshop." If you so desire to see it that way, your relationship is like living in an ongoing personal growth workshop designed specifically for you.

14

Integrating Your Transformation

Throughout human history people have been weavers. Knit into the artistry of their tapestries are stories, history, family lore, healing, and love. Weaving is an art form as well as a hobby and a vocation. Some take to it naturally, while others need many lessons and lots of guidance.

The journey of postpartum is a process of knitting yourself back together—weaving the tapestry of your life. At first, all the threads on the loom of your life are colored by the experience of birth, new parenthood, and your baby. The threads of your former life may not be visible, so consuming are the early days of parenthood. Keep weaving your breaths into moments, your moments into days, your days into weeks, and your weeks into months. You don't make it to your baby's first birthday all in one stretch. You arrive there by knitting shorter segments of time into longer ones, weaving threads together into a row, then a section, and eventually—a tapestry.

GATHERING THE THREADS OF YOUR TAPESTRY

In early postpartum, it is common to want to reach into your basket of threads for the familiar colors—vibrant or mellow—of your former, pre-baby life. You want to begin weaving them in right away, anxious to return to your former self. Instead, remember you are a weaver, an artisan, crafting the tapestry of your *life*. In order to make a beautiful and complex tapestry, one best appreciated from a distance rather than up close, the weaver must not rush to integrate a thread before its time.

Sometimes, the thread needed in your tapestry is buried under the ones on top . . . under the ones catching your attention and begging to be used. As the weaver of your life, you might have to pause and reflect, dig beneath what is obvious, and sometimes go looking for an entirely new ball of thread. Sometimes you have to cut a thread that used to be vitally important to your life design, but now no longer fits. While there are patterns you can follow, no two tapestries are ever the same. It is often the places where a thread bulges or puckers that gives the tapestry its unique beauty and artistry. It is how the tapestry is brought to life that makes it special, and ultimately, an heirloom.

Joy

What brings you joy? Have you asked yourself this question lately? Do you know the answer? It can be difficult to bring joy into your life if you don't know what is truly joyful to you. Pay attention to what brought you joy prenatally as well as what brings it to you now, in new parenthood. Try shifting your attention from what doesn't bring you joy to what does. Changing what you're looking for can inform your behavior. Remember the personal question exercise in chapter 10 . . . look out the front windshield toward what you want more of in your life so you can do what's needed to help make that your reality.

Sometimes a whisper of who you are shows up as the inspiration to pick up a creative project you started before birth or perhaps as a new endeavor that reminds you of your former passion. In the first year of my parenting journey, I met a woman in my baby group who was a badass paralegal before her first baby was born. Jennifer could research anything. *Anything*. She and her partner decided she would stay home with their baby. Motherhood did not require much of Jennifer's amazing intellect. At some point in the first year of her child's life, Jennifer became the entire neighborhood's resource for information. She would research any information we new parents needed—from the best sunscreen to the safest car seats—compiling data about value, health and environmental impacts, and efficacy. Jennifer found a bit of herself in those research projects and integrated them into her new identity as a parent. The rest of our baby group loved having access to Jennifer's research!

To begin finding your way back to yourself, try bringing your attention to one thing you loved before you were a parent . . . something that brought you joy.

Before our first child was born, my husband and I bought a home. It had zero curb appeal, and I often laugh when I remember buying it as it was so ugly! What could we have seen in it? For me, it was a blank slate upon which we could create our home. Before I became pregnant, I took pottery classes, I continued a daily yoga practice, and I was obsessed with nurseries. I loved to go to nurseries and wander the aisles touching and smelling all the different plants. Perennials were my favorite. After my first son was born, my 6:00 a.m. yoga practice became impossible, and pottery classes and work both required childcare, which I didn't have. But gardening . . . that was my savior. I could wander the nurseries with my baby in tow and touch, smell, and gaze at all the plants, buying one or two as I slowly brought life to our garden. One plant at a time, I found my way back to something I loved.

Gardening became part of my spiritual practice within motherhood. In fact, my dear friend and I nicknamed our favorite nursery the "Temple of Plants." Tending my garden was a daily ritual and visiting the Temple of Plants was like going to a house of worship. As my kids grew, I planted and tended a kitchen garden we could all enjoy. In it I built a sandbox and playhouse so the kids could play while I put my hands in the earth. Until my kids were about four and six years old, the garden was the best place for me to simultaneously parent and tend to my own inner landscape. My kitchen garden was a thing of beauty, but more than that, it was my personal salvation.

Another mother I worked with, Kate, is a costume designer. Her identity was deeply connected with her career. When she had her son, her career took a backseat for a bit since when she worked, she would become so completely absorbed with the project that nothing else existed. She couldn't imagine doing that while parenting a baby. At a couple of months postpartum, she began making the most amazing outfits and costumes for her son. I mean, these were spectacular! A little while after that, she picked up a small job that she thought she could navigate without complete absorption. And sometime after that, she took a bigger job. She basically stitched threads together until her worlds and passions were integrated.

What small part of your life can you weave into your world as a parent? Is there an intellectual pursuit, a creative passion, or a beloved career that will help you remember you're *you* as well as a parent?

Some new parents find themselves through solitary exploration. Reading, prayer, meditation, or cooking can be ways to find joy. Activities of this sort often have to take on new qualities postbaby—meditation might be a few conscious breaths on the toilet if no other options are possible! Maybe your joy is finding a way to return to something physical like yoga, running, or hiking. I found that my yoga practice had to change, drastically, after years of regularity and dedication. But getting back into my body was essential for my wellbeing. To tend to that need, I would push a stroller or wear my baby and go for a hike.

Walking is often a balm to a new parent's soul. Find a nice-enough path or road and get outside, weather permitting. Maybe there are parent meetups at a nearby park or parent-and-me exercise classes for a dose of bodily connection and community. Remember that early postpartum is not the time to force yourself back to a highly demanding exercise routine. Force has no place in postpartum.

There is no one right way to reconnect with yourself. Explore. Experiment. Make mistakes. Try again. Open to what brings you joy *as a parent* . . . it might be something completely different than you anticipated prenatally. Be open to the possibility that what calls to you as a parent and what's possible as a parent might be very different from what called to you as an individual before baby. Be creative, resourceful, and ask for help. Your well-being matters.

Your Body

If you have grown and birthed a baby from your body, it is common to feel distant from the sensual and sexually vibrant person you may have been before. This distance is a normal part of the natural impulse to turn inward often associated with new parenthood and postpartum. And as you return to fullness, one of the threads of your former self you might eventually want to find and weave with again is your connection to yourself as a sexual being. But where to begin?

The Pelvic Floor

Pregnancy, labor, and birth require a lot from the pelvic floor muscles, and the strain can lead to difficulties long after the postpartum period. Find out if your insurance will cover a visit to a pelvic floor physical therapist or a pelvic floor specialist and get referrals. I highly recommend that everyone who has given birth vaginally or surgically see a pelvic floor specialist. Under their guidance you can bring your pelvic floor back to full health and vitality following birth. This should be a regular part of postpartum care available to everyone.[1]

Opening to Your Body's Changes

Your body has been changed by birth. Whether you birthed vaginally or abdominally, your body bears the marks of the experience within its tissue. Before you can return to a sexual relationship with another, you will likely need to reconnect with your physical body *personally*. The process of sexual reconnection can be like meeting someone for the first time even though they have somehow been connected with you forever. It can be foreign, scary, exciting, triggering, and multifaceted.

To begin the process of returning to yourself as a sexual being, it can be helpful to reacquaint yourself with your body. The following exercises can help.

Try This

Looking in the Mirror

Light a candle and/or adjust the lighting, put on special music, or mark sacred space in another way that works for you and your environment. Try standing naked in front of a full-length mirror (if you don't have one, you can use a smaller mirror). Scan your body with a soft gaze and a kind inner voice. Let your eyes float over all of the parts of your body that you can see, both front and back. Notice the changes like they were those a tree undergoes with the changing seasons. Practice gazing without preferences. Instead use the eyes of an observer, taking it all in. What do you notice is new, different, or changed? Keep breathing.

If you are ready to go further, continue on. Using a hand mirror, look at your labia, and spreading the labia, look into your vagina. What do you see? What is new or unfamiliar about this special area now that you've had a baby?

Reflect on the experience. You can journal or just take a moment to think about what you noticed. What arises for you as a result of this exercise? Who is the person you see in the mirror? What do you love about your body? Where is it strong? Where is it soft? What is your favorite part of your new parent body?

Close this exercise ritually by blowing out the candle or taking a mindful breath. Be sure to mark the shift from sacred space back to everyday life.

Postpartum Body Poems

I give new parents in my postpartum groups the exercise to write a poem about their body. Try it using this format: *This is my (body part). It (what it does for you now as a mother/parent).* Or, for plural parts like eyes, ears, hands, etc.: *These are my _____, they _____.*

Be sure to include your reproductive/sexual parts (breasts, belly, vagina, and/or labia) as well as a few others of your choice. If you gave birth surgically, be sure to include your scar. Identify at least eight body parts. As you write, let your thoughts roam over the areas of your body. What do you know about your belly now that is new or different? How have your eyes changed now that they look at your child and see the world as a parent? Do not shy away from the tricky, painful, or disappointed feelings. Your poem is to be a truthful expression of your exploration of your body as a parent. It won't likely be all shining praise and glory. It will likely be complex and varied. Let yourself reflect with courage and curiosity. You might be surprised by what you learn about yourself.

Here's a poem written by a new mom as part of one of my postpartum circles for inspiration.

This is my hair,

> my sword and shield, sickle and wheat. Now reborn a lifeline, rope swing, a kite string that tethers tiny hands to a grounded ship. A lightning rod in the sand, an anchor.

These are my shoulders,

> boulders and landslide alike, knotted with the ropey lines of The Future, missteps, catastrophe, death, of small and frightful whispers in the night. The machines that lift joy into the air as bright as the sun, laughter widening the breath of the room. Hiked up at once with the gravity of worry and the privilege of bliss.

These are my breasts,

> once empty and yet too round, too low, too much. Reliably inescapable, they blushed with the punchline of avoidance. Now they are burning with nourishment, heavy against my ribcage, an overflowing river for a tiny, wild mouth, hungry for the world, humming along the button of a nipple. They have been sung into life.

These are my hands,

> long like yours, long like my mother's, fine-combed lifelines and blue river veins. Tools of a soft trade. A patchwork quilt of a before and an after, pillowing feather-soft hair and catching sinews of drool with steel string calloused fingertips, busy like birds.

This is my belly,

> forever-shadow. Once ashamed and purposeless, it became resolute—bursting with intent, convex and smooth and brave and brooding with the weight of an ocean. Now a bundle of ribbons, rippled, an aching emptiness that is still too full, bound and bound again, soft and drunk on an unbearable lightness.

These are my hips,

> ajar, widened—like a jaw, bones bruised against the bed, steering the ship while sinking beneath the daily ritual. The battered fulcrum, the broad base of a sleepy, hiccupping metronome.

This is my vagina,

> split open like the earth, like the bright moon pinned so low in the sky, a tree

branch bowing, heavy with fruit. This is the alchemy and miracle, the invisible
freight train of strength, the pliant and supple center of power. Lying dormant
through this season. The scarred, the cloaked, the hidden away and quiet queen.
This is my heart,
a drum machine birthed from my body, a tiny hummingbird feeding on the sage
in the backyard.

Anna[2]

If you'd like to read a few more of these poems written by parents
who have participated in my postpartum groups, go to my blog at
brittabushnell.com/blog.

I know your time is limited and adding something to your already busy
schedule might make you grimace, but this exercise is a profound one. I
recommend you write your body poem and then read it to someone who
can receive it with depth and tenderness. The process of sharing is another
vulnerable and powerful experience toward knowing yourself anew.

Reconnecting with Your Senses

Early parenthood can be overwhelming to the senses. From the myriad
of new smells that arrive with a newborn to the amount of time new
parents spend in physical contact with another human being, the
senses can flood, shut down, and close off. In order to reconnect with
yourself as a sensual being, you have to allow yourself to *feel* again as a
person not only as a parent.

Try This

Taking a Ritual Bath

This exercise, given to me by my former teacher Sofia Diaz many years ago,
is the one I share with my postpartum groups to enhance reconnection
with the senses. It involves taking a sacred and ritualized bath (or a
shower if you don't have access to a tub). But don't put down this book and
immediately go jump in the tub. Wait. There's more to it than that. The
purpose of this bath is to enliven your senses and to connect to your body as
an autonomous being with desires and sensations beyond those associated

with parenthood. It's meant to be both ritualized and romantic. This is sacred time for you.

Carefully select items to stimulate all of the senses—sight, hearing, touch, smell, and taste—prior to actually taking the bath. Is there a special oil, soap, or other bath additive whose texture and scent make you happy? How about music that helps you relax and a candle or special lighting that helps set the mood for a reverent and romantic event? Is there a beverage or a sweet morsel that enlivens your sense of taste? Give attention to all of the senses. Be sure to schedule your bath after your baby goes to sleep or ask someone else to care for your baby so that you won't be disturbed for *at least 30 minutes*.

Once you have gathered all the elements of your ritual bath and carved out time to give to it, then you're ready. Run the water to a pleasing temperature, and set up the space with reverence in mind. This is *your* time to give to your body and your senses, yours and yours alone.

Climb in. Settle your body into the water. Expand your awareness, noticing the sights, smells, and sounds in the room. Close your eyes and

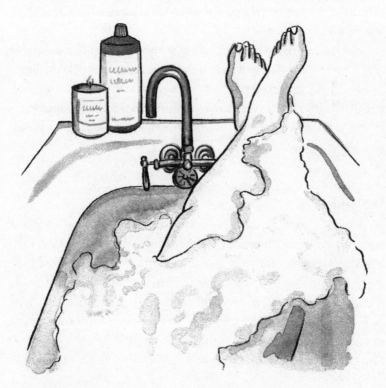

feel whatever you feel. Try slowing your breath and heart rate as you settle your nervous system and drop slowly into your body more and more. Don't be surprised if your mind gets active. It is common for the mind to hum when the body slows. If this happens, gently bring your attention back to the sensual stimulation in the room—the smells, sounds, and the rhythm of your breath.

Bring your awareness to the water on your skin. Run your hands over your arms and feel the touch. Add your legs and feet, then your torso, chest, shoulders, neck, face, and head. Gently touch your whole body with your eyes closed.

Then open your eyes and explore your body visually. Scan your body from top to bottom with a tender gaze. Be sure to keep breathing.

Take a sip of the beverage or a bite of the sweet morsel you selected. Savor the taste in your mouth. Bring your full awareness to the sensations on your taste buds. Take your time.

You can address the senses in whatever order inspires you. Don't worry about doing anything in a particular way. Simply bring your awareness to each of the five senses and your breath over the course of the bath. This is *your* time with *your* body.

When you are done with your bath or shower, dry off and sit on your bed or in a comfortable chair and journal about the experience (if journaling isn't your thing, call a friend with whom you can share the experience verbally). Lastly, close up the sacred space you created by blowing out candles or taking a mindful breath, consciously ending your bathing ritual before reengaging with your normal activity.

Sexual Being

We discussed sex a bit in the previous chapter, but that was specifically regarding sex as an element of your romantic relationship. Here I wish to address sexuality for your sake. Many of us have been raised believing that sexual arousal is something shared with a partner. I believe that being sexually alive and vibrant is everyone's birthright. While each of us has a unique baseline of sexual energy, everyone deserves to feel sexual vibrancy pulsing through their bodies and brains. For many new parents, accessing arousal is difficult. You might be touched out, tired, and disconnected from passion, your partner, and your own body. Even the *idea* of sex can be hard to get excited about. If you want to reconnect with desire and increase your interest in sex, there are things you can do.

I am a sexually vibrant person. I like to feel myself aroused both physically and mentally, regardless of whether or not my partner is with me. When that aliveness has waned at different times in my life, I've missed it. Early parenthood was one such time. It was important to me to bring my sexual vitality back to life, not just to be able to share it with my husband, but for me.

The key doorway for me is my body, but my mind has always been the initial gatekeeper that occasionally needs to be reminded that I like sexual energy moving through my body! After having a baby and once I was ready to feel sexual again, I started paying attention to what ignited even the tiniest spark of sexual openness or interest. I became aware that romantic movies that opened my heart were great for this. At first it wasn't sexy movies that helped; those were too direct for my postpartum brain. All I needed was to be inspired to *feel* more. Reading and listening to audiobooks had a similar effect. What media I ingested mattered. When I watched more violent movies, documentaries, or even the news, or when I read self-help books rather than heartful fiction, my connection to my libido waned. In this regard, my brain played a starring role in reconnecting to sexual desire.

Once my mind remembered that sexual interest was something *I* desired, I had to remind my body how to feel. I started with the sensual touch exercises I shared in the previous chapter as well as the bathing exercise from this chapter. Then, I incorporated more embodied practice. When I moved, danced, or exercised . . . really anything that reminded me that I was a person with a body, it helped. At one point, when my kids were little, I made cooking dinner a regular dance-party boogie. I'd turn up music I loved and moved, boogied, and danced my way through dinner preparations. Practices of this sort helped bring me back slowly to a level of sexual vibrancy.

In addition, I used self-pleasuring practices to remind my body what it felt like to be aroused. Bringing myself to climax alone before sharing my sexuality with my husband was necessary. I needed to find out what an orgasm as a mother felt like, and how it was and wasn't different after giving birth. The more I marinated my body and brain in practices that supported arousal, the more sexually vibrant I became. Like so many aspects of what I've shared in this book, tending to my sexual vibrancy became part of my regular practice. I share my sexual passion with my husband when it works for both of us, but I maintain it for myself.

What helps you connect to desire? Begin to notice even the smallest sparks of interest. Pay attention to what opens you to sexual energy or even the idea of becoming aroused. Maybe nature, art, physical activity, touch, stories, massage, yoga, good conversation with your partner, outings with friends, dancing, taking baths, or something else opens you a little bit. Notice what works. Then, do more of that as part of your personal practice. It's up to you whether or not you share any of this with your partner. Your practice is for you.

Reengaging with the World

For most parents, there comes a time when it becomes necessary (whether financially or for mental well-being) to reengage with the world outside of your home. Sharing your gifts with others takes many forms: returning to work or school, engaging in creative expression, athletic pursuits, volunteer work, or spiritual practices, or even having a fulfilling social life that does not involve your child. While these differ in many ways, they often share the reality of leaving your child with someone else and, as such, share some emotional similarities as well.

Guilt

For many parents, leaving their child for any reason brings up guilt and feelings of not doing enough for their baby. Returning to work can be particularly guilt inspiring, especially if you have to return before you feel emotionally and physically ready. Guilt is a huge issue for modern parents trying to do so much. The voice that fuels guilt tends to begin with "I should" or "I shouldn't." I know for myself, guilt surfaces around ideas of not doing enough for my children or my career. These two passions make demands on limited time and energy.

Choices have to be made. Navigating the feelings such decisions raise is a normal part of the personal practice of parenthood.

I work with feelings of guilt by using the seven reminders I shared for working with parenthood as a personal practice in chapter 12. Number seven, "nurture a kind inner voice," is especially helpful. When the inner voices that fuel the feelings of guilt get loud, I have to get quiet and speak tenderly to myself. My most helpful self-talk goes something like this: "Of course you wish you could do it all. It's normal to feel these desires conflicting with each other. You can only do what you can do. It's okay to feel sad about _____." I had to speak with this kind inner voice as I focused on writing this book while my younger son faced new challenges without me there to support him. Practicing the kind inner voice soothed my feelings of guilt and helped me return my energy to the choice I made to put my career first in this moment.

Guilt does not go away, but it can be worked with and soothed. Developing these tools will serve you as you step away from 24/7 parenting and reenter the world still going on around you.

Shame

Guilt's partner is often shame. Pay attention to the voices of guilt and attend to them kindly, for they have a way of morphing into shame. You can tell the difference when your action no longer causes a feeling of guilt about what you did but transforms into a statement about your worth as a person or parent. Shame in parenting is common. When you hear yourself think or say, "I'm a bad mom" or "I'm a bad dad," you're in the realm of shame.

There are lots of things that feed shame: staying quiet about feelings and partaking in comparison are two big ones that can trigger shame for me. If I see myself slipping into a shame spiral, there is a good chance I've been quiet or comparing myself to others. What helps me pull out of a shame spiral is to share my feelings with someone I trust and who doesn't believe the story I'm telling myself. Not all people can offer this kind of support or be a safe space to share. Really the only response that doesn't help is someone telling me they have no idea what I'm talking about. That response only fuels shame! Share your shame story with an empathetic listener or become one for yourself by deepening the practice of kind self-talk.

Anxiety

In addition to guilt and shame, the voices of "should" can trigger anxious thoughts of what could happen if you aren't able to do everything yourself. Trusting others to care for your child or your work projects is not always easy. Guilt fuels anxiety, and then anxiety drives more guilt. It can be a vicious cycle. Again, use the tools from chapter 12 to support you in unhooking from this destructive thought chain. If your anxiety gets to the point where you can't ease out of it on your own, seek professional help.

Financial Concerns

Becoming a parent usually comes with added financial stress. There are more expenses and often reduced income. What an awful combo! Sadly, many parents spend a good portion of their salary covering childcare. Some parents don't see the point of going back to work when the net gain is so low, while others depend on the differential between salary and childcare no matter how small. There are many factors that go into decisions around childcare and work. Like all things about parenting, there is no one right way for everyone. The good news is, children are resilient. My kids' preschool teacher, Linda, had a saying that has stuck with me for years: "What kids get, they come to expect. What they expect, they come to need." This simple phrase is brilliant. Make decisions that work for you, and your children will not only adjust, they will come to expect and need it that way.

Time Pressure

Money is not the only resource in limited supply for new parents. Time also seems to be increasingly tight, as you step back into the world by either returning to work or attending to a passion or pursuit. Get help where and how you are able. How might you alleviate some of your time pressure?

A mom I know found the time pressure to be real, and trying to get everything done only led to more guilt and struggle. She had to create firm boundaries around her work time and family time. While at work, she focused on work. When at home, she turned off her computer and muted her phone so she could be fully present with her family. The time pressure actually inspired her to be more efficient with her time and hold firmer boundaries.

Other parents find themselves burning the midnight oil to finish things that didn't fit into the number of waking hours divided between work and family. As someone who has mostly worked for myself and from home, creating boundaries has been critical to my emotional well-being.

Additionally, in our highly connected technological age, it is sometimes our availability to others that puts the squeeze on our time. Be thoughtful and intentional about how you use your devices and what does and doesn't feed your soul. For some parents, social media is what keeps them sane as a parent. For others, social media, texts, and emails are distractions that take them away from what truly feeds their soul. Our family made a "no phones at the table" rule that has helped us stay connected during precious time. Check in with yourself and create a habit of making thoughtful choices about when and how you engage with technology.

Partnership

A study released in December 2017 showed that even as women catch up to men as family earners, and actually outpace them in academic achievement, they continue to bear a disproportionate portion of household and family responsibilities.[3] If you are in a relationship and are co-parenting, you don't have to do this alone. Share the tasks that fill your days. Just as children adapt to how things are done, so, too, do partners. If you try to do it all, the expectation will develop that that's just how your family operates. Establish habits that share the load of tasks that come with being an adult, such as bill paying and taxes, as well as household chores and childcare responsibilities.

My career has been a wonderful catalyst for creating opportunities for my husband to solo parent our kids. When I traveled to teach workshops when our kids were three and five, my husband would be alone with them for three to seven days. During those work trips, he had to do everything for them, from shopping and cooking to putting them to bed and getting them to preschool. Our kids developed a deep trust in their dad's ability to emotionally and practically care for them. Their trust deepened my trust and helped soothe any pangs of guilt creeping in from being away. I believe my kids are more resilient as a result of their ability to rely on either of their parents for support.

Relief

One of the side effects of returning to work or spending more time away from your baby that many parents don't expect is *relief*! It can simply feel divine to have time without your child! Some parents find that returning to work is a joyful change from the boredom and nonstop demands that frequently fill days alone with a baby. Relief is as normal as guilt and sometimes they come hand in hand! It's okay to feel relief. Parenting is hard. Taking time away from your baby is healthy for everyone. Enjoy what you can, when you can!

KEEP WEAVING

This process of weaving yourself back together is not to be rushed. Not all threads of all textures and colors will belong. You need to gather and sort, select and discard. You're making a tapestry that is uniquely yours.

In weaving, there are the threads that stay more or less in place and that give the tapestry its structure. These make up the "warp." In our lives, the warp represents the unchanging parts of our beingness that give our unique life a type of continuity year to year even as the events, people, and places change. That's not to say that the warp never breaks, but rather that those threads rarely change.

For me, one of the threads of my warp is a type of determination that has always been part of me. My first nickname given to me as a baby just as I learned to crawl was "Bulldozer" (oh, my poor parents!). To this day, there is still some bulldozer within me. It has tempered and mellowed, giving more space to the other vehicles on the road of my life, but much of that gritty girl, Bulldozer, still resides within the warp of my life's tapestry . . . even in my hardest moments.

Another warp thread that gives my tapestry structure is my playful goofiness. I take all things very seriously (that's the bulldozer), including my willingness to be goofy and make fun of myself in the service of connection. It is this part of me that showed up as a preschool teacher as well as a birthday party clown. Another thread has been my commitment to always be growing.

You, too, have warp threads that give structure to the tapestry you're always weaving. What are some of your core elements—those warp threads—that give stability to your life even when it's in flux?

Woven under and over the vertical warp threads are the horizontal threads, or the "weft," that give the tapestry its color, variety, and pattern. The weft changes frequently in our lives depending on what we face, the people with whom we associate, our pursuits, and our passions. For example, my relationship to yoga has been a dominant weft in my life tapestry for many years, fading during early postpartum and again after a skiing accident that required major knee surgery, but although it faded and brightened, it was always visible. My passion for working with people around birth has been another weft for about twenty years, and parenthood has had a few different threads going for about that same amount of time.

While the horizontal threads that give my tapestry color and design change over time, the warp stays more or less the same. When I had a

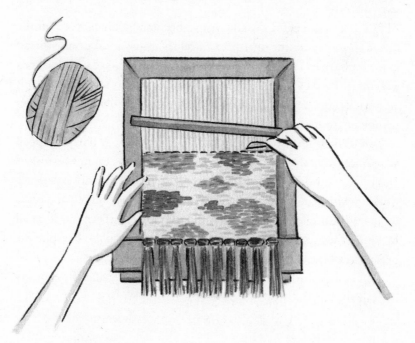

new baby for the first time, parenting consumed the weft of my weaving, but the structure of my tapestry was held together for better or worse by my doggedness—the Bulldozer—as well as the clown and the growth threads of my warp. My love of family (an heirloom from my grandmothers) is another warp thread in my life's tapestry that can be seen throughout my life, including my home life and profession.

Reflect on your personal tapestry. Identify some of the threads of who you are that give your life stability even in the midst of change and upheaval. What is true about you even when external events are in flux? Come up with at least a few. Write them down in a journal or on a piece of paper or, if you are really inspired, make a piece of art that incorporates your words in a visual way. Regardless of how you put these threads into visual form, place them where you can easily see and be reminded of these unchanging qualities of who you are. Once you've done that, dive a bit deeper.

Think, write, or discuss with a friend or with your partner about how those parts of you might help during this transformative time of new parenthood. How might they give structure and stability to your tapestry during a time when the weft strings are moving and changing so frequently?

Life is ever-changing. While we can become highly focused on the thread in our hand, the one we're currently using, it is but one thread in the tapestry of a life. If you make a mistake or a thread buckles, keep weaving. Mistakes have a way of becoming the artistry of the work. Step back, look at your creation. Myopia tends to obscure the bigger picture of the masterpiece in the making.

Thread by thread you are creating your life anew. It doesn't happen all at once. It is, after all, a creative endeavor, and art cannot be rushed. This profound work of the soul may take a lifetime. From my experience working with parents for the past twenty years, birthing a baby often catapults the need to do so into prominence. You have been transformed by birth. The experience of becoming a parent may guide or inspire the personal work you are called to do for many years to come.

Remember through it all: you are a weaver, crafting the tapestry of your life.

Epilogue

Becoming a parent is a wild and transformative journey!

Expect many experiences along the path of parenthood but do not expect to get it "right." No such utopian destination exists in reality. Instead, expect to have moments of profound joy as well as intense boredom. Expect to lose your patience and be amazed by just how much you actually have. Expect to laugh and cry harder than you ever have before. Expect to lose your shit over little things, as well as big. Expect to be surprised by what you didn't know and couldn't know ahead of time. Expect to have moments where the love you feel for your child catches you by surprise as well as moments when you wonder, "Who is this kid?"

By the time you get to this phase in your parenting journey, you will have crossed a most significant threshold, lost or discarded aids you previously thought indispensable, borne witness to the metamorphosis of your identity, and brought a one-of-a-kind human being into this world.

It is my hope that you have grown along the way, not into some perfect parental version of yourself, but into someone who embraces their imperfections with humility and humor. May you learn to be open to the unbidden while traversing the wild and unpredictable landscape that is birth and parenthood. May you gain the maturity to know that rough moments happen and develop resilience to navigate them. May you foster a kind inner voice and the ability to decipher the whisper of your unique wisdom even when it sounds uncertain. May you find or build a community of people with whom you can share the journey of parenthood and also be nurtured while you grow as a parent and a person.

While I don't know you personally, I have great faith that you have done and continue to do your absolute best every step of the way, even when you make "mistakes." I believe that you deserve kindness, support, and encouragement now and as you walk forward, embracing your beloveds, into the often brutal, imperfect, and magical journey we call parenthood.

Acknowledgments

Turning my doctoral dissertation into this book was like laboring to birth a baby. I have had to face many gateways of doubt, let go of control, push even when I was exhausted, and lean on others for help. Birthing this book has taken a team!

I must begin my acknowledgments thanking all the courageous, dedicated, and loving parents I have had the great honor to mentor. A special thank you to those who have allowed me to share their stories, words, or poetry: Katrina and Jesse, Neela and Tom, Becca, Theresa, Emily, Anna, Sharon and Billy, Vanessa, Cathlene and Jeff, Brandy, Zoe and Jamie, Alice and Max, Natalie, Katherine, Kate, Alissa, Jennifer, Rosie, Gus and Emily, and Amanda and Dennis.

I am forever indebted to Pam England, my mentor and guide in the field of childbirth. It is through many years of learning, sharing, partnership, and friendship that this work is even possible. I am profoundly grateful for Pam's support and her encouragement that I share practices and stories first learned from her.

Special gratitude goes to my agents, Michele Martin and Steve Harris. Their understanding of my message and faith in me came at a pivotal time, and their support and guidance have been invaluable throughout this long labor. And thank you to my dedicated editor, Diana Ventimiglia, and the rest of the amazing Sounds True team including Lauren Slawson, Jeff Mack, and Christine Day, as well as Tami Simon for her support of my book. Also to Nikki Van De Car at kn literary for her editorial eye early in the process. Deep gratitude to my talented illustrators, Meghann Stephenson and Amy Haderer at [M]otherboard. Thank you also to my gifted photographers and clients, Steven Kreps and Anna Elledge.

Profound gratitude for the community created at YogaWorks in the 1990s. Especially to Chuck Miller, Maty Ezraty, and Lisa Walford for being my teachers, Shiva Rea for inviting me to model the second trimester poses in her prenatal video (twenty years ago), and Seane Corn for being a role model of strength and purpose to this day. To my many other extraordinary teachers and guides outside of birth work—Michaela Boehm, Sofia Diaz, Dr. Clarissa Pinkola Estés, Tsoknyi Rinpoche, Jack Zimmerman, Pattabhi Jois, Sharath Jois, David Lynch, Teri Pichot, Jean Shinoda Bolen, Lewis Mehl-Medrona, Hari Grebler, Linda Hinrichs, Jeff Lough, Christine Carter, Geffen Rothe, and Dr. Jay Gordon. And to my stellar dissertation committee: Chris Downing, Jacqueline Feather, and Ronald L. Grimes, whose support of my research ultimately led to the publication of this book.

My work in birth has been supported by an amazing community of colleagues. Thank you to Kathie Neff, Brandy Ferner, Rebecca Coursey, and Cindi Cnop, my friends and colleagues in the truest sense of the words; to Lori Bregman, my "book doula" and Topanga soul sister; to midwives Sara Howard and Sarah Obermeyer, who read my manuscript and offered valuable feedback and support; to Virginia Bobro, my former business partner, cofacilitator, and friend; and to those who influence my work in ways both known and unknown—Kimberly Ann Johnson, Emily Wannenburg, Ana Paula Markel, Kimberly Durdin, Yana Katzap-Nackman, Becca Gordon, Haize Hawke, Kate Zachary, Rena Sassi, Nkem Ndefo, Patti Quintero, Aleksandra Evanguelidi, Elliot Berlin, Margo Kennedy, Haley Oaks, Leslie Stewart, Penny Simkin, Christine Morton, Phyllis Klaus, Robbie Davis-Floyd, Jen Kamel, Adriana Lozada, and many others. Thank you also to my Birthing From Within community then and now including—Joanna Nightengale, Sarah Juliusson, Barb Steppe, Erika Primozich, Deidre Coutsoumpos, Rosanna Davis, and Nicole Morales.

Deepest gratitude to Carrie for her irreplaceable friendship and partnership on the parenting path, to each family of the Topanga

Baby Group for treasured community, to Tracy and Adam for a depth of friendship hard to find, to Katie and Nicole for sharing women's wisdom, depth, and love, to each of the "Wild Women," and to Patrick and Melissa, who offered support in numerous and profound ways. Thank you also to my Hawaii-based family, especially Karin, Mimsy, Denise, Tora, Sari, and Iam. And thank you to Alecia Moore for her continued support and endorsement of my work years after taking my class. I am profoundly grateful.

Love and gratitude to my remarkable extended family for their love and support, including my siblings by blood or marriage—Alissa, Brent, Tyler, Gavin, Neela, Dylan, Wyatt, Amanda, Dennis, Jeff, Tom, Molly, Maggie, Kate, Justin, and Jodi—my growing number of nieces and nephews, especially the five I've watched make their entrance into the world; my beloved goddaughter, Aleksa, for providing me the opportunity to mother a daughter and supporting me in the production of this book (as well as so much more!); and my many fathers—Nolan, Louis, Colin, Rob, and Ben. In particular, I wish to thank my mothers: my mother-in-law (mama), Marilyn, for her steadfast faith in my abilities, my stepmom, Nancy, for initiating eight-year-old me into the wonders of childbirth, and to my mother, Paula, for planting seeds of mythology and ritual in my heart early on and for teaching me about life, being a woman, and parenting.

I wish to thank my children, Kaden and Rumiah, who made me a mom and called me to be the best mother I could be. They have cheered me on throughout this process, even when it took me away from doing something fun as a family. They have been my most profound teachers, and being their mother is an immense honor. Watching them fly off into the future of their creation fills me with hope and joy.

And to my husband, Brent, whose faith in my ability surpassed my own. It was his commitment to and support of my work that not only made writing possible but kept me going when I was most doubtful. I am profoundly grateful to have a life partner who shares a fundamental dedication to growth. He is the banks to my river.

Notes

Introduction: No Right Way to Birth

1. Except where identifiers were used all names are those of real people who have given me permission to share their stories.

Chapter 1: Birth as a Meaning-Making Experience

1. Arnold van Gennep, *The Rites of Passage*, trans. Monika B. Vizedom and Gabrielle L. Caffee (Chicago: University of Chicago Press, 1960).

2. Bruce Lincoln, *Emerging from the Chrysalis* (Oxford, UK: Oxford University Press, 1981).

3. Brené Brown, *Rising Strong* (New York: Random House, 2015).

4. Daniel H. Pink, *A Whole New Mind: Why Right-Brainers Will Rule the Future* (New York: Penguin, 2005), 103.

5. Jonathan Gottschall, *The Storytelling Animal: How Stories Make Us Human* (New York: First Mariner, 2013), 67.

6. John Medina, *Brain Rules: 12 Principles for Surviving and Thriving at Work, Home, and School* (Seattle, WA: Pear Press, 2014).

7. Paul J. Zak, "Why Your Brain Loves Good Storytelling," *Harvard Business Review*, November 05, 2014, accessed October 28, 2018, hbr.org/2014/10/why-your-brain-loves-good-storytelling.

8. Pink, *Whole New Mind*, 101.

9. Doug Stevenson, "Storytelling and Brain Science: This Is Your Brain on Story," Association for Talent Development, July 26, 2016,

accessed October 28, 2018, td.org/insights
/storytelling-and-brain-science-this-is-your-brain-on-story.

10. Paul J. Zak, "How Stories Change the Brain," *Greater Good Magazine*,
December 17, 2013, accessed October 29, 2018, greatergood
.berkeley.edu/article/item/how_stories_change_brain.

11. Gordon H. Bower, "Mood and Memory," Semantic Scholar, January
01, 1981, accessed October 29, 2018, semanticscholar.org/paper
/Mood-and-memory.-Bower/895d2af2765ff94dfcc5f72a9d48588b8
6c960f5.

Chapter 2: Start Where You Are

1. "Safe Prevention of the Primary Cesarean Delivery," *American
Journal of Obstetrics and Gynecology*, 210.3 (March 2014), ACOG
(website), accessed January 30, 2019, acog.org/Clinical
-Guidance-and-Publications/Obstetric-Care-Consensus-Series
/Safe-Prevention-of-the-Primary-Cesarean-Delivery.

2. "State of the World's Mothers 2013: Surviving the First Day," Save
the Children, 2013, savethechildren.org/content/dam/usa/reports
/advocacy/sowm/sowm-2013.pdf.

Chapter 3: Prepare to Be Unprepared

1. Michael J. Sandel, "The Case Against Perfection," *Atlantic* (website),
April 2004, theatlantic.com/magazine/archive/2004/04
/the-case-against-perfection/302927/.

2. Eugene R. Declercq, et al. *Listening to Mothers III: Pregnancy and
Birth* (New York: Childbirth Connection, 2013), 14.

3. Declercq, *Listening to Mothers*, 15.

4. Michael Blastland and A. W. Dilnot, *The Numbers Game: The
Commonsense Guide to Understanding Numbers in the News, in Politics,
and in Life* (New York: Gotham Books, 2010), 64.

5. Yvonne Bohn, Allison Hill, and Alane Park, *The Mommy Docs'
Ultimate Guide to Pregnancy and Birth* (Cambridge, MA: Da Capo,
2011), 101.

6. Rebecca Dekker, "The Evidence on: Due Dates," Evidence Based Birth,
April 15, 2015, accessed October 18, 2017, evidencebasedbirth.com
/evidence-on-inducing-labor-for-going-past-your-due-date/.

7. Ben Rabinovich, "Meghan Markle Pregnant: When Is the Royal Baby Due?," *Daily Mail*, October 15, 2018, accessed May 20, 2019, dailymail.co.uk/news/article-6277483/Meghan-Markle-pregnant -Royal-baby-due.html.

8. *Merriam-Webster's Dictionary*, (2015), s.v. "plan."

9. S. H. Deering, J. Zaret, and A. J. Satin, "Patients Presenting with Birth Plans: A Case-Control Study of Delivery Outcomes," *Journal of Reproductive Medicine* 52, no. 10 (October 1, 2007): 884–87, accessed January 30, 2019, europepmc.org/abstract/med/17977160.

10. R. Grant, A. Sueda, B. Kaneshiro, "Expert Opinion vs. Patient Perception of Obstetrical Outcomes in Laboring Women with Birth Plans" *The Journal of Reproductive Medicine* 55, no. 1–2 (January 1, 2010): 31–35, europepmc.org/abstract/med/20337205.

11. Neel Shah, "Hospital Management Practices May Put Women at Risk for C-Sections, Complications During Childbirth," press release, Harvard School of Public Health (website), July 11, 2017, accessed January 30, 2019, hsph.harvard.edu/news/press-releases /hospital-management-practices-cesareans/.

Chapter 4: Too Much Information!

1. Rebecca Dekker, "Premature Rupture of Membranes," Evidence Based Birth, updated on July 10, 2017, accessed on January 29, 2019, evidencebasedbirth.com/evidence-inducing-labor-water-breaks-term/.

2. P. M. Dunn, "John Braxton Hicks (1823–97) and Painless Uterine Contractions," *Archives of Disease in Childhood—Fetal and Neonatal Edition* 81, no. 2 (September 1999): 157–58, accessed May 16, 2019, doi:10.1136/fn.81.2.f157.

3. To learn more about the World-Wide Labyrinth Locator, visit labyrinthlocator.com.

4. "Safe Prevention of the Primary Cesarean Delivery," *American Journal of Obstetrics and Gynecology* (March 2014) ACOG (website), accessed January 2, 2019, acog.org/Clinical -Guidance-and-Publications/Obstetric-Care-Consensus-Series /Safe-Prevention-of-the-Primary-Cesarean-Delivery.

5. Phyllis L. Brodsky, *The Control of Childbirth: Women Versus Medicine Through the Ages* (Jefferson, NC: McFarland, 2008).

6. Rebecca Dekker, "Friedman's Curve and Failure to Progress: A Leading Cause of Unplanned Cesareans," Evidence Based

Birth, updated April 26, 2017, accessed January 30, 2019, evidencebasedbirth.com/friedmans-curve-and-failure-to-progress-a -leading-cause-of-unplanned-c-sections/.

7. "Asaro," Jimmy Nelson (website), accessed January 30, 2019, jimmynelson.com/people/asaro.

Chapter 5: Into the Wilderness

1. Online Etymology Dictionary, s.v. "lochia (n.)," accessed January 16, 2019, etymonline.com/word/lochia.

2. W. K. C. Guthrie, *The Greeks and Their Gods* (Boston: Beacon Press, 1955), 71.

3. Louann Brizendine, *The Female Brain* (New York: Harmony Books, 2007), 100.

4. Brizendine, *Female Brain*, 99.

5. Brizendine, 100.

6. Marie Prevost, et al., "Oxytocin in Pregnancy and the Postpartum: Relations to Labor and Its Management," *Frontiers in Public Health* 2 (January 27, 2014), doi:10.3389/fpubh.2014.00001.

7. Aleeca F. Bell, Elise N. Erickson, and C. Sue Carter, "Beyond Labor: The Role of Natural and Synthetic Oxytocin in the Transition to Motherhood," *Journal of Midwifery & Women's Health* 59, no. 1 (2014): 35–42, accessed October 31, 2018, doi:10.1111 /jmwh.12182.

8. Prevost, "Oxytocin in Pregnancy."

9. Anna-Riitta Fuchs, et al., "Oxytocin Receptors in the Human Uterus During Pregnancy and Parturition," *American Journal of Obstetrics and Gynecology* 150, no. 6 (1984): 734–41, accessed October 31, 2018, doi:10.1016/0002-9378(84)90677-x.

10. Online Etymology Dictionary, s.v. "endorphin (n.)," accessed October 31, 2018, etymonline.com/word/endorphin.

11. Pam England and Rob Horowitz, *Birthing from Within: An Extra-Ordinary Guide to Childbirth Preparation* (Albuquerque, NM: Partera Press, 1998), 180.

12. Paul J. Zak, *The Moral Molecule: How Trust Works* (New York: Dutton, 2012), 64.

13. England, *Birthing from Within*, 6.

Chapter 6: The Four-Letter Word

1. Naomi Wolf, *Misconceptions: Truth, Lies, and the Unexpected on the Journey to Motherhood* (New York: Doubleday, 2001), 184.

2. Thank you to my friend and colleague Nicole Morales for this Harry Potter/birth connection.

3. J. K. Rowling, *Harry Potter and the Sorcerer's Stone* (Waterville, ME: Thorndike Press, 1999), 298.

4. Grantly Dick-Read, *Childbirth Without Fear*, 4th ed. (London: Pinter, 2013), 18–20.

5. Maggie Nelson, *The Argonauts* (Minneapolis, MN: Graywolf Press, 2015), 124.

Chapter 7: Partners on the Journey to Birth

1. I'm grateful to my friend and colleague Rebecca Coursey for this nuanced instruction.

2. See Gena Kirby's website at genakirby.net.

Chapter 8: Someone's Parent

1. Albert R. Jonsen, Mark Siegler, William J. Winslade, *Clinical Ethics: A Practical Approach to Ethical Decisions in Clinical Medicine*, 8th ed. (New York: McGraw-Hill, 2015), 57.

2. "Ethical Decision Making in Obstetrics and Gynecology," ACOG Committee Opinion Number 390, American College of Obstetricians and Gynecologists, December 2007, accessed January 30, 2019, doi: 10.1016/0738-3991(91)90076-H.

3. This building-a-bridge process was inspired by the one Pam England describes in *Our Birthing from Within Keepsake Journal* (Albuquerque, NM: Birthing From Within Books, 2003).

4. Neel Shah "Hospital Management Practices May Put Women at Risk for C-Sections, Complications During Childbirth," press release, July 11, 2017, accessed January 30, 2019, hsph.harvard.edu/news /press-releases/hospital-management-practices-cesareans/.

5. Miriam Greenspan, *Healing Through the Dark Emotions: The Wisdom of Grief, Fear, and Despair* (Boulder: Shambhala, 2004), 37.

Chapter 9: What Happens in the Cocoon

1. "Achievements in Public Health, 1900–1999: Healthier Mothers and Babies," CDC (website), October 1, 1999, accessed January 24, 2019, cdc.gov/MMWR/preview/mmwrhtml/mm4838a2.htm.

2. "Reproductive Health: Pregnancy Mortality Surveillance System," CDC (website), August 7, 2018, accessed January 19, 2019, cdc .gov/reproductivehealth/maternalinfanthealth/pregnancy-mortality -surveillance-system.htm; "Reproductive Health: Infant Mortality," CDC (website), August 3, 2018, accessed January 19, 2019, cdc.gov /reproductivehealth/maternalinfanthealth/infantmortality.htm.

3. While the story of Inanna is ancient and of Sumerian origin, the idea to use this myth for childbirth preparation, as well as many of the links connecting the story to modern-day childbirth, I got from Pam England. I am grateful that she has encouraged me to share it far and wide. While I take liberties with some of the details, crafting them to my use, the general story comes from *Inanna: Queen of Heaven and Earth* (New York: Harper, 1983), the collaborative product of Assyriologist Samuel Noah Kramer (who translated the cuneiform) and storyteller Diane Wolkstein (who crafted the translation into poetry modern readers might enjoy).

4. Paul Collins, "The Sumerian Goddess Inanna (3400–2200 BC)," *Papers from the Institute of Archaeology* 5, 103–118, accessed January 30, 2019, doi: 10.5334/pia.57.

5. Joshua J. Mark, "Sumer," Ancient History Encyclopedia, April 28, 2011, accessed October 18, 2017, ancient.eu/sumer/.

Chapter 10: You Do Not Have to Be Perfect

1. Michael J. Sandel, "The Case Against Perfection," *Atlantic* (website), April 2004, theatlantic.com/magazine/archive/2004/04 /the-case-against-perfection/302927/.

2. Roberts Avens, *The New Gnosis: Heidegger, Hillman, and Angels* (Putnam, CT: Spring Publications, 2003), 97.

3. Ovid, *The Metamorphoses of Ovid*, trans. Allen Mandelbaum (San Diego, CA: Harcourt, 1993).

4. To explore it more deeply I recommend reading Taigen Dan Leighton's *Zen Questions: Zazen, Dogen and the Spirit of Creative Inquiry.*

5. "WHO Statement on Caesarean Section Rates," World Health Organization, April 2015, accessed January 24, 2019, doi: 10.1111/1471-0528.13526.

6. Niall McCarthy, "Which Countries Conduct the Most Caesarean Sections?" Statista, January 13, 2016, accessed January 25, 2019, statista.com/chart/4221/which-countries-conduct-the-most -caesarean-sections/; David Smith, "Caesarean Section Rates in South Africa 'recklessly High,' Warn Experts," *Guardian*, September 24, 2014, accessed January 25, 2019, theguardian.com/world/2014 /sep/24/caesarean-section-south-africa.

7. "WHO Statement on Caesarean Section Rates," World Health Organization.

8. "Guidelines and Evaluation Criteria for Facilities Seeking Baby-Friendly Designation," Baby-Friendly USA, July 16, 2018, babyfriendlyusa.org/wp-content/uploads/2018/10/GEC2016 _v2-180716.pdf.

9. Karen Maezen Miller, *Momma Zen: Walking the Crooked Path of Motherhood* (Boston: Trumpeter Publishers, 2007), 21.

Chapter 11: The Early Days of Parenthood

1. Adriana Lozada (the Birthful Podcast host) has a great postpartum plan document that you can download from her website at birthful .com/postpartumplan/.

2. Two good options to make organizing a meal train easier are mealtrain.com and mealbaby.com.

3. Postpartum Support International at postpartum.net is a good resource.

4. Heng Ou, et al. *The First Forty Days: The Essential Art of Nourishing the New Mother* (New York: Abrams, 2016), 25–28.

5. Thank you Geffen Rothe for your valuable coaching and guidance. This instruction clearly stuck with me!

6. Peter A. Levine, *Waking the Tiger: Healing Trauma* (Berkeley: North Atlantic Books, 1997), 162.

7. Levine, *Waking the Tiger*, 10, 261.

8. Information on Birth Story Listeners can be found at birthingfromwithin.com/birth-story-listening/.

9. Miriam Greenspan, *Healing Through the Dark Emotions: The Wisdom of Grief, Fear, and Despair* (Boulder: Shambhala, 2004), 45.

10. Jean Shinoda Bolen, *Artemis: The Indomitable Spirit in Everywoman* (San Francisco: Conari, 2014), 69.

11. Betty De Shong Meador, *Uncursing the Dark: Treasures from the Underworld* (Wilmette, IL: Chiron Publications, 1992), 107.

Chapter 12: Transformed Parenthood

1. George Loewenstein, "The Psychology of Curiosity: A Review and Reinterpretation," *Psychological Bulletin* 116, no. 1 (1994): 75–98, accessed January 30, 2019, doi:10.1037//0033-2909.116.1.75.

2. I am indebted to Teri Pichot of Denver Center for Solution-Focused Brief Therapy for her guidance in teaching me almost all of what I know about using a solution-focused mind-set with parents. This work has changed my life.

3. Part of this section was originally written as a blog shared on my website, brittabushnell.com/the-myth-of-self-care.

4. I'm grateful to my former teacher Sofia Diaz for this piece of eternal wisdom.

5. Pema Chödrön, *Start Where You Are: A Guide to Compassionate Living* (Boulder: Shambhala, 2018), 14.

Chapter 13: Couples Who Are Parents

1. John Mordechai Gottman and Julie Schwartz Gottman, *And Baby Makes Three: The Six-Step Plan for Preserving Marital Intimacy and Rekindling Romance after Baby Arrives* (New York: Three Rivers Press, 2007); Alyson Fearnley Shapiro, John M. Gottman, and Sybil Carrère, "The Baby and the Marriage: Identifying Factors That Buffer Against Decline in Marital Satisfaction after the First Baby Arrives," *Journal of Family Psychology* 14, no. 1 (2000): 59–70, doi: 10.1037//0893-3200.14.1.9.

2. Matthew D. Johnson, *Great Myths of Intimate Relationships: Dating, Sex, and Marriage* (Malden, MA: John Wiley and Sons, 2016), 123.

3. Casie Leigh Lukes and Aviva Romm, "The Truth about Postpartum Hormones and Healing: A Q&A with Aviva Romm, MD," *Experience Life*, January 17, 2018, accessed January 28, 2019, experiencelife.com/article/postpartum-hormones/.

4. Brent and I are grateful to Jack Zimmerman, one of our teachers at the Ojai Foundation, for this relationship-enriching concept.

5. John M. Gottman, Julie S. Gottman, Carolyn Pirak, and Joni Parthemer, *Bringing Baby Home: Couple's Workbook* (Seattle, WA: Gottman Institute, 2014), 25.

6. I am forever grateful to Jack Zimmerman and the other teachers at the Ojai Foundation for teaching us this practice, which has become one of the ritual cornerstones of my marriage and family life.

7. Lewis Mehl-Medrona and Barbara Mainguy, "Introducing Healing Circles and Talking Circles into Primary Care," NCBI, spring 2014, accessed January 24, 2019, doi: 10.7812/TPP/13-104.

8. I'm grateful to Lewis Mehl-Medrona for his guidance around how to share this practice respectfully.

9. Jack M. Zimmerman and Virginia Coyle, *The Way of Council* (Las Vegas: Bramble Books, 1996), 28–35.

10. Gottman, *Bringing Baby Home*, 133.

Chapter 14: Integrating Your Transformation

1. For more on the pelvic floor and postpartum recovery, read Kimberly Ann Johnson's book, *The Fourth Trimester*.

2. I'm grateful to Anna V. for sharing this profound piece of self-reflective poetry.

3. "New Research Shows the 'Mental Load' Is Real and Significantly Impacts Working Mothers Both at Home and Work," Bright Horizons Family Solutions, December 20, 2017, accessed January 25, 2019, brighthorizons.com/newsroom /mental-load-impact-working-mothers-study.

Index

classes/childbirth classes, 48, 66

cocoon phase of transformation, 15–16, 153–54

communication practices, 128–29, 241–46

contractions, 66–68, 78–79
 ice "contractions," 101–4, 107

control
 desire for, 30–32, 174
 birth plan, 40–45
 and certainty, 173–74
 due dates, 36–40
 opening to the unbidden, 32–35
 pain, 111–12
 perfection, 174–75

darkness, 83

death
 childbirth and infant mortality, 155
 denial of death, 154
 The Descent of Inanna, 156–68, 170–72, 180, 212, 280n3 (chap. 9)
 identity death, 168–69
 rebirth, 169–72

Dekker, Rebecca, 37

The Descent of Inanna, 156–68, 170–72, 180, 212, 280n3 (chap. 9)

Dick-Read, Grantly, 97

dilation, 57–59, 63, 66

doctors. *See* health-care professionals

doulas, 134, 136–37

due dates, 36–40

effacement, 59

emotions, 88–91

endorphins, 78–80

England, Pam, 5–6, 51, 56, 80, 91, 177, 280n3 (chap. 9)

epidurals, 109–10, 181–84

exceptionalism, 175–76

exercises. *See* "Try This" exercises

expectations, 69

family (extended family), 204–7, 246–47

fear, 91, 147–51

feedback, 128–29

"focus" during labor, 104–5

forgiveness (self-forgiveness as a parent), 223–24

The Fourth Trimester (Johnson), 208, 283n1

Friedman's curve, 66

the future, 177

gender inclusivity, 7

Gottman, John and Julie, 236, 246

Gottschall, Jonathan, 18

Greenspan, Miriam, 148, 210

guilt, 262–63

Healing Through the Dark Emotions (Greenspan), 148

health-care professionals
 B.R.A.I.N. decision-making tool, 145
 choosing provider and birth location, 146–47
 communicating with, 142–44
 consent and refusal, 141–42
 informed decision-making, 144–46

help. *See* support

Hicks, John Braxton, 54

hormones, 19–20, 76–80
 endorphins, 78–80
 fear, 91
 stress, 88–91

hubris, 176

humility, 174, 177

hypothalamus, 81

ideals (cultural ideals), 25

Inanna, 156–68, 170–72, 180, 212, 280n3 (chap. 9)

independence, glorification of, 115–16

inducing labor, 34, 77

initiation rites, 12

innocence, 139

intentions (birth intentions), 42–44

involution, 207

Permissions

Excerpt(s) from *A Whole New Mind: Why Right-Brainers Will Rule the Future* by Daniel H. Pink, copyright © 2005, 2006 by Daniel H. Pink. Used by permission of Riverhead, an imprint of Penguin Publishing Group, a division of Penguin Random House LLC. All rights reserved.

Excerpt(s) from *The Moral Molecule: The Source of Love and Prosperity* by Paul J. Zak, copyright © 2012 by Paul J. Zak. Used by permission of Dutton, an imprint of Penguin Publishing Group, a division of Penguin Random House LLC. All rights reserved.

Excerpt(s) from Doug Stevenson, "Storytelling and Brain Science: This Is Your Brain on Story," Copyright © 2016 Doug Stevenson. Used with permission. www.storytelling-in-business.com.

Excerpt(s) from the article "The Case Against Perfection" by Michael Sandel. Copyright © 2004 by Michael Sandel. Used with permission from The *Atlantic*. www.theatlantic.com/magazine/archive/2004/04/the-case-against-perfection/302927/.

Excerpt from *Listening to Mothers Survey III* ©National Partnership for Women & Families. Used with permission. Source: www.nationalpartnership.org/listeningtomothers.

About the Author

Dr. Britta Bushnell is a childbirth, relationship, and parenthood specialist, author, and speaker. For the past two decades, she has taught classes to midwives, doctors, rock stars, Hollywood celebrities, and thousands of other parents in preparation for birth. Britta blends her personal and professional experience in the childbearing year with her doctoral study in mythology and psychology, bringing a fresh approach to an age-old human experience. She is an engaging teacher, storyteller, and speaker, and whether she's addressing a room of expectant parents, new mothers, kids, or seasoned birth professionals, she has a way of captivating and inspiring them all.

Britta lives in Southern California with her husband, Brent, and (when they are in town) their two sons, who are now young adults.

About Sounds True

Sounds True is a multimedia publisher whose mission is to inspire and support personal transformation and spiritual awakening. Founded in 1985 and located in Boulder, Colorado, we work with many of the leading spiritual teachers, thinkers, healers, and visionary artists of our time. We strive with every title to preserve the essential "living wisdom" of the author or artist. It is our goal to create products that not only provide information to a reader or listener, but that also embody the quality of a wisdom transmission.

For those seeking genuine transformation, Sounds True is your trusted partner. At SoundsTrue.com you will find a wealth of free resources to support your journey, including exclusive weekly audio interviews, free downloads, interactive learning tools, and other special savings on all our titles.

To learn more, please visit SoundsTrue.com/freegifts or call us toll-free at 800.333.9185.

In loving memory of Beth Skelley, book designer extraordinaire. Her spirit lives on in our books and in our hearts.

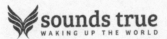